Ultrasound-guided Musculoskeletal Procedures

Luca Maria Sconfienza
Davide Orlandi • Enzo Silvestri
Editors

Ultrasound-guided Musculoskeletal Procedures

The Lower Limb

Springer

Editors
Luca Maria Sconfienza
Unit of Radiology
IRCCS Policlinico San Donato
San Donato Milanese, Milano
Italy

Department of Biomedical Sciences
for Health
Università degli Studi di Milano
Milano
Italy

Davide Orlandi
Department of Internal Medicine
Università degli studi di Genova
Genova
Italy

Enzo Silvestri
Ospedale Evangelico Internazionale
Unit of Radiology
Genova
Italy

ISBN 978-88-470-5763-0 ISBN 978-88-470-5764-7 (eBook)
DOI 10.1007/978-88-470-5764-7

Library of Congress Control Number: 2015947819

Springer Milan Heidelberg New York Dordrecht London

Printed on acid-free paper

Springer-Verlag Italia Srl. is part of Springer Science+Business Media (www.springer.com)

Foreword

The success encountered by the previous book entitled *Ultrasound-Guided Musculoskeletal Procedures: The Upper Limb* witnessed the great interest of our colleagues for ultrasonography of the musculoskeletal system and for the related ultrasound-guided treatments. Thus, we propose this second book, devoted to ultrasound-guided procedures to treat common and less common pathology of the lower limb.

Some therapeutic procedures, such as hip viscosupplementation, received a great impulsion from the use of ultrasound guidance and currently represent one of the central procedures that can be used to treat hip osteoarthritis, mainly to delay total hip replacement. In the hip, ultrasound guidance is also very useful to treat periarticular pathologic conditions, such as gluteal, rectus femoris, and hamstring enthesopathy or iliopsoas bursitis.

The knee has always been regarded as an "easy" joint that could be treated without any imaging guidance. However, ultrasound has been shown to improve needle placement accuracy, especially in obese people in whom anatomical references are poor, or in those patients affected by inflammatory or degenerative disease, which need a highly targeted treatment. Compression neuropathies around the knee have also been addressed.

In the ankle, this book has been focused on the treatment of common diseases, such as plantar fasciitis, Morton's neuroma, and periarticular ganglia, including the principal indications to treatment, the most convenient access routes, and the drugs to use.

In conclusion, this book represents a comprehensive and practical guide to perform ultrasound-guided procedures of the musculoskeletal system in the lower limb, both for beginners, who want to learn the basic principles, and expert physicians, who want to implement new procedures in their clinical practice. The procedures here reported derive mostly from the long-lasting experience of our musculoskeletal interventional team and are only in small part derived from literature, as evidence on large samples still missing in some diseases. We also acknowledge the effort of our younger colleagues in this volume, whose invaluable contribution revealed to be an excellent asset.

Pietra Ligure, Italy
May 2015

Giovanni Serafini, MD

Contents

Part III The Ankle

Part IV The Foot

Contributors

Alice Arcidiacono Postgraduate School in Radiodiagnostics, University of Genova, School of Medicine, Genova, Italy

Angelo Corazza Postgraduate School in Radiodiagnostics, University of Genova, School of Medicine, Genova, Italy

Emanuele Fabbro Unit of Radiology, Ospedale Santa Corona, ASL 2 Savonese, Pietra Ligure, Italy

Giulio Ferrero Unit of Radiology, Ospedale Santa Corona, ASL 2 Savonese, Pietra Ligure, Italy

Francesca Lacelli Unit of Radiology, Ospedale Santa Corona, ASL 2 Savonese, Pietra Ligure, Italy

Carmelo Messina Postgraduate School in Radiodiagnostics, University of Milano, School of Medicine, Milano, Italy

Davide Orlandi Department of Internal Medicine, University of Genova, Genova, Italy

Silvia Perugin Bernardi Postgraduate School in Radiodiagnostics, University of Genoa, School of Medicine, Genova, Italy

Riccardo Sartoris Postgraduate School in Radiodiagnostics, University of Genoa, School of Medicine, Genova, Italy

Luca Maria Sconfienza Unit of Radiology, IRCCS Policlinico San Donato, Milano, Italy

Department of Biomedical Sciences for Health, University of Milano, Milano, Italy

Giovanni Serafini Unit of Radiology, Ospedale Santa Corona, ASL 2 Savonese, Pietra Ligure, Italy

Enzo Silvestri Unit of Radiology, Ospedale Evangelico Internazionale, Genova, Italy

General Aspects of US-Guided Musculoskeletal Procedures

1

Luca Maria Sconfienza, Davide Orlandi, Carmelo Messina, and Enzo Silvestri

Ultrasonography (US) is a quick and noninvasive imaging modality that allows for the precise visualization of most soft tissue components of the musculoskeletal system. Providing real-time imaging, this modality also enables accurate guidance during interventional procedures, thus reducing to minimum the risks of complications. As US is considered a relatively operator-dependent modality, a strict scanning technique is mandatory to obtain the best outcome possible. If clinical knowledge is the basic requirement for any diagnostic or therapeutic process, then US-guided interventional procedures analogously require thorough knowledge of the equipment being used. Also good technical skills are needed in order to extract the maximum amount of information that can be obtained with the available equipment, while avoiding the numerous pitfalls and artifacts of this imaging modality.

L.M. Sconfienza (✉)
Unit of Radiology, IRCCS Policlinico San Donato, Milan, Italy

Department of Biomedical Sciences for Health, University of Milano, Milano, Italy
e-mail: io@lucasconfienza.it

D. Orlandi
Department of Internal Medicine, University of Genova, Genova, Italy
e-mail: theabo@libero.it

C. Messina
Postgraduate School in Radiodiagnostics, University of Milano, School of Medicine, Milan, Italy
e-mail: carmelomessina.md@gmail.com

E. Silvestri
Unit of Radiology, Ospedale Evangelico Internazionale, Genoa, Italy
e-mail: silvi.enzo@gmail.com

Setting

Room

As far as possible, a specific room should be devoted to interventional procedures. This is due to the fact that the room should be kept as clean as possible. Also, proper setting for the room used in the interventional procedures is a prerequisite in ensuring high safety standards together with a smooth workflow.

The general requirements should be:

Structure

- The rooms and spaces are related to the nature and extent of the activities performed. The minimum clearance should be 4 m, with a 1.5-m clearance around the bed.
- Area of observation
- Medical staff preparation area
- Storage area for clean material
- Disposal area for soiled material
- Waiting area
- Toilet and sink for patients
- Toilet and sink for medical staff

L.M. Sconfienza et al. (eds.), *Ultrasound-guided Musculoskeletal Procedures: The Lower Limb*, DOI 10.1007/978-88-470-5764-7_1

Technical Equipments

- Adjustable (height and angular adjustments) surgical bed
- Ventilation system capable of maintaining a constant air cleaning within the room
- Adjustable lighting system illuminating the surgical field
- Medical gas pipeline systems
- Emergency trolley
- Emergency call system

US System

While choosing the right US system can be extremely challenging, an informed and useful choice is more likely if the purchaser has a clear concept of the US-guided interventional procedures that will be performed. In general, high-level systems may be needed in a diagnostic setting, while interventional procedures may be performed also with basic US systems.

In general, the basic requirements for dedicated interventional US equipment are:

Ergonomics

- System size and steering: the system should be portable or movable, allowing for transportation to remote clinics or for operating-theater work. Machines used regularly for mobile work should be robust and easy to move. Handheld portable machines are an option.
- Moveable (swivel and tilt) monitor and control panel, including height adjustment for different operators and situations.
- Keyboard design facilitating access to the required functions, without the need for stretching or twisting.

Materials

- Long-lasting materials with high resistance to common antiseptics
- Smooth surfaces that can be easily and quickly cleaned

Technical Requirements

- Quick probe selection and switching process, possibility of connecting several probes
- Dynamic frequency capability
- Dynamic focusing control, number, and pattern of focal zones
- Advanced functions such as beam steering, sector angle adjustment, and zoom

Probes

- A high-frequency linear-array probe is needed for most procedures regarding superficial soft tissues (10/12 MHz or higher)
- A convex probe (1–6 MHz) may be needed to perform procedures in deeper locations (such as hip joint)
- Compatibility with US guidance devices
- Ergonomic handle shape to preserve a neutral wrist position
- Probe design allowing use with either hand

US-Guided Procedures

Prior to any interventional procedure, a preliminary US evaluation of the affected site should be performed to confirm the pathology to treat and to plan carefully the procedure. This is of paramount importance as the patient's condition may have changed since the previous examination.

Clinical History

Basic information on the patient's medical history should be collected. A brief preliminary talk, covering the following items, should be held with the patient or his/her physician:

- Present complaint(s)
- History of the present complaint(s)
- Past medical history
- Drug/allergy history
- Family medical history

- Personal and social history
- Systems review

In general, the three most urgent considerations that must be carefully assessed before any US-guided interventional procedure are:

- Blood-thinning pathologies or the use of blood-thinning drugs: in general, antiplatelet therapy is not a contraindication to soft tissue procedures. Anticoagulant therapy is not usually a contraindication for most procedures performed with fine needles. However, we usually ask patients to switch to antiplatelet therapy 5 days prior treatment.
- Drug allergies: although uncommon, some people may be allergic to anesthetic drugs. It is worth asking for any prior allergic event during any dental procedure involving anesthesia.
- Diabetes: the use of steroid in diabetic patients has been proven to minimally increase glycemia, although this variation is generally not clinically significant. However, please note that these patients may be more prone to develop local infections. Thus, extra caution should be taken to maintain sterility at the highest level possible. Also, antibiotic prophylaxis may be administered (we occasionally use amoxicillin 875 mg + clavulanic acid 125 mg twice a day per 6 days).

Explanation of Contraindications to the Interventional Procedure and Informed Consent

Despite the minimal invasiveness of the interventional procedures described in this book, the patient must be provided with an accurate explanation of the possible contraindications related to the planned procedure. Although the complication rate associated with these procedures is extremely low, patients should be aware that their occurrence cannot be ruled out entirely. The subjects that must be clearly explained to the patient are the following:

- Discomfort during the procedure
- Discomfort after the procedure and the possibility of steroid-related flare
- Potential risk of infection
- Potential risk of tendon rupture

After receiving this information, the patient must formally agree to the procedure by providing both verbal and written informed consent. We prefer to use different consent forms for each procedure, in which the procedure is clearly explained on the same sheet that is signed by the patient.

Antisepsis

All US-guided interventional procedures must be performed with aseptic techniques in order to avoid any risk of contamination by infectious organisms (bacteria, fungi, viruses) or other disease-causing microorganisms.

The cornerstones of a safe US-guided interventional procedure are:

- Antisepsis: transient microorganisms are removed from the skin using chemical solutions for disinfection.
- Aseptic non-touch technique: it minimizes the risk of infection by ensuring that only uncontaminated objects/fluids make contact with sterile/susceptible sites. The only part of the sterile equipment that may be handled is that which will not be exposed to the susceptible site. Reusable equipment employed during an aseptic procedure should be cleaned with wipes and must be fit for purpose. All packs/single-use equipment, e.g., dressing packs, cannula packs, and syringe packs, must be intact, with a still-valid expiration date, and without visible signs of contamination.
- Operator sterility: accurate and effective hand hygiene is the most important component of good infection prevention and control, given that the hands are a common route of infection transmission. Transient bacteria can be removed by effective hand hygiene techniques, e.g., by washing the hands with an antimicrobial liquid soap and water or by using an alcohol-based hand rub. Sterile gloves are mandatory.
- Probe antisepsis: the US probe and probe wire are swiped with dedicated antiseptic solutions. A sterile probe cover may also be used.

- Patient antisepsis: the skin cannot be "sterilized", but certain chemical preparations reduce microbial levels. Our antisepsis procedure is composed of a first step in which a brown water-based povidone-iodine solution is used to mark the treated area, and after 1–3 min (sufficient to let the antiseptic act), in the second step, a transparent solution of 70 % isopropyl alcohol and 2 % chlorhexidine is applied. This allows for both doubling disinfection of the skin and not staining the US probe during procedure.
- Surgical field: draping of the treating area may be extremely helpful, especially for longer procedures. Adhesive tissues can be used for this purpose.
- US contact gel: conventional US contact gel should not be used for aseptic US-guided procedures. Contact gel is not usually needed for shorter procedures, as both probe and skin are wet due to antiseptic solutions. For longer procedures, sterile contact gel can be used.

Needles and Syringes

The wide range of different interventional procedures implies the use of different kinds of needles.

Needles of different diameter (measured in gauges, G; the lower the number, the higher the diameter) and length (measured in millimeters) can be used. In general, conventional 5-, 10-, and 20-ml syringes carry 20–21 G, 5-cm-long needles that can be used for most purposes:

- Very superficial procedures in a sensitive area can be performed using thin (26–32 G) and short (2 cm) needles.
- Procedures that require the aspiration of dense collections, such as ganglions or hematomas, are performed using larger (14–16 G) needles. Needle length is strictly related to target depth.
- Spinal needles are used for deep locations such as hip joints or in obese patients. The most common spinal needles used in these procedures are 9–12 cm and 18–22 G.

There are different types of syringe in respect to luer design. For most procedures, we prefer to use syringes with slip, eccentric luer, as they can be easily connected and disconnected to the needle. Syringes come with a number of designs for the area where the blade locks to the syringe body. Few procedures (e.g., hyaluronic acid injection) may require higher pressures; thus, the use of luer-lok syringes may be advisable. Syringe capacity varies according to the amount of fluid to inject or to drain.

For the most common upper limb procedures, we recommend the following:

- 1–2 ml: used around the ankle/foot for intermetatarsal bursitis injections, for Morton's neuroma treatment and for the treatment of tenosynovitis
- 5–10 ml: used to inject trochanteric and retrocalcaneal bursitis and to drain small collections and for platelet-rich plasma injections
- 20 ml: used for calcification lavage and aspiration or the evacuation of fluid collections

How Is the Needle Inserted?

Guidance of the needle under US can be performed with either the lateral or coaxial approach. In the former, the needle is kept perpendicular to the US beam and is inserted on the short side of the probe. In the latter, the needle is inserted on the long side of the probe, parallel to the US beam. The lateral approach has the advantage of excellent visibility of the needle, which, however, crosses a larger amount of tissue before reaching the target than is the case with the coaxial approach (Fig. 1.1a). On the other hand, the coaxial approach is burdened by a reduced needle visibility, but it can be used when the space around the target is greatly restricted. In this latter case, however, adequate experience is needed to achieve satisfactory results (Fig. 1.1b).

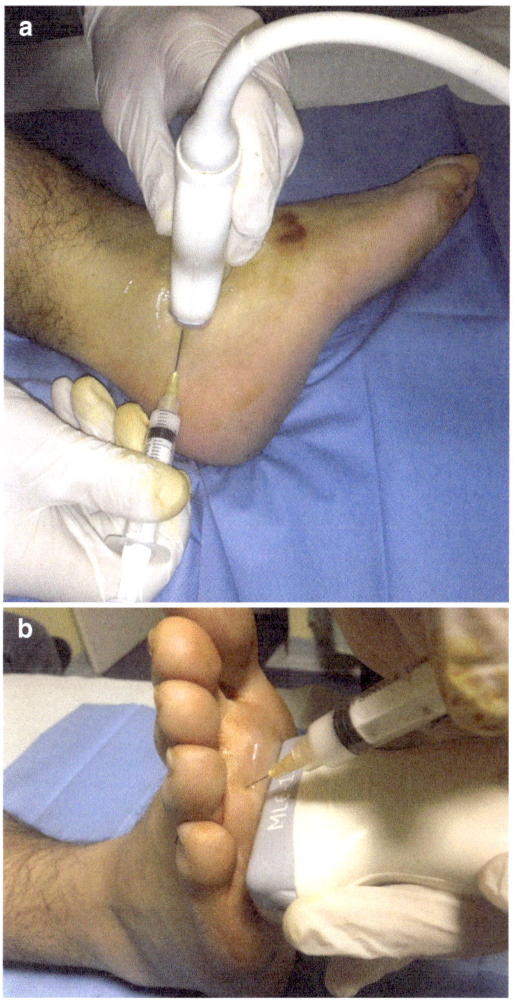

Fig. 1.1 (**a**) With US-guided lateral approach, the needle is inserted on the short side of the probe allowing for an excellent visibility. (**b**) With US-guided coaxial approach, the needle is inserted on the long side of the probe, allowing for a reduced path in soft tissues but visibility is limited only to the tip

Drugs

Local Anesthetics

US-guided interventional procedures may require local anesthesia to minimize pain and discomfort. The type and amount of anesthetic used depends largely on the procedure itself and the involved anatomical location.

The effect of local anesthetics is given by their ability of interrupting neural conduction, by inhibiting the sodium channels. In most cases, this inhibitory activity follows their diffusion through the neural membrane into the axoplasm, where they enter sodium channels. The local anesthetic molecule consists of three different components, the combination of them giving specific properties to the molecule. The lipid solubility of the compound enhances diffusion through both nerve sheaths and the neural membranes of the individual axons comprising a nerve trunk. This property correlates with drug power, as the higher the liposolubility, the greater portion of drug enters neurons.

Fast-acting local anesthetics, such as a 2 % lidocaine solution, are injected with a small needle around and within the area to be treated. Patients will initially experience a brief stinging sensation related to the needle and the anesthetic being introduced; bicarbonate buffering significantly reduces this type of sensation. We use a mixture of one part of bicarbonate every four parts of anesthetic. Within seconds, typically, the area becomes numb. Lidocaine solutions are also an option for US-guided diagnostic nerve blocks, with the anesthetic injected around the nerve over the level of the suspected pathology.

Long-acting local anesthetics, such as a 0.25 % bupivacaine hydrochloride solution, are injected in association with corticosteroids for local relief at sites of musculoskeletal discomfort (articular and extra-articular) and for therapeutic nerve blocks.

Permanent side effects are extremely uncommon provided that maximum doses are respected. Temporary effects may be experienced by patients that may include:

- Numbness of the tongue
- Dizziness
- Blurred vision
- Muscle twitching

Local anesthetics depress the central nervous system dose dependently. A maximum dose of 20-ml 2 % lidocaine can be considered safe and more than sufficient for most local musculoskeletal procedures.

Some patients may claim that they are allergic to local anesthetics. Upon careful questioning, however, it becomes clearer that they experienced vagal reactions related to the injection procedure or cardiac palpitations attributed to epinephrine either contained in the solution or released endogenously. Although rare, allergic reactions to local anesthetics have been reported in the scientific literature, but in none of these cases was there a confirmed IgE-mediated hypersensitivity reaction. Nevertheless, patients have occasionally experienced symptoms consistent with an allergic reaction to amide local anesthetics. Usually, asking patients whether they had ever experienced any problems with dental anesthesia is a reliable diagnostic test.

Corticosteroids

Inflammation is one of the body's first reactions to injury. Increase in local blood flow transports polymorphonuclear leukocytes, macrophages, and plasma proteins to the injured area, where arteriolar flow is redistributed thus producing stasis and hypoxia at the injury site. The resulting infiltration of the affected tissues by leukocytes, plasma proteins, and fluid causes the redness, swelling, and pain that are the typical features of inflammation.

In the musculoskeletal system, different causes of inflammation can be found, including arthritis, tenosynovitis, bursitis, and trauma. It has also been shown that inflammation is present in other diseases that have been traditionally regarded as degenerative, such as osteoarthritis.

In degenerative/overload tendinopathy, no inflammatory cells are usually seen. However, angiofibroblastic proliferation can be frequently seen.

Steroid action includes series of different mechanisms that act by limiting capillary dilatation and the permeability of the vascular structures. These drugs restrict the accumulation of polymorphonuclear leukocytes and macrophages, reduce the release of vasoactive kinins, and inhibit the release of destructive enzymes that attack the injury debris and destroy normal tissue indiscriminately.

Steroids are normally produced by the human body. However, in daily practice we commonly use synthetic molecules that can be adapted to the clinical needs. Synthetic drugs used in clinical practice are normally derivatives of prednisolone. All have anti-inflammatory potencies per dose unit that are somewhat greater than that of cortisol.

Commercially available preparations can be either soluble or insoluble. In the musculoskeletal system, low-soluble preparations are preferably used. The main advantage of these preparations is that they require hydrolysis by cellular esterases to release the active principle: thus, their action in the joint is long-lasting. Other soluble preparations can also be used, such as dexamethasone-based drugs. The advantages of these preparations are that they are taken up rapidly by cells and thus have a quicker onset of effect but with a concomitant reduced duration of action.

The duration of action of corticosteroids can be estimated based on their biologic half-life, pharmaceutical half-life, or duration of clinical benefit. While the duration of clinical benefit is the most practical assessment, it really represents a very subjective parameter and differs widely in literature reports, without statistically significant differences.

Corticosteroids can also be mixed with other drugs (e.g., anesthetics, hyaluronic acid) in the same syringe. The indications and the concentration of such mixtures are however quite confusing in literature, and they are mainly based on personal experience.

The established adverse effects associated with corticosteroid injections may include infection, cutaneous flares, local fatty atrophy, skin depigmentation, tendon rupture, and increased blood glucose level.

Infection is one potential complication of all invasive maneuvers. However, using a good sterile technique, the incidence of this complication seems to be negligible. Note that local steroid injection may decrease local immunity thus potentially favoring the development of infections. The most common adverse event is cutaneous flare, which is a local increase in inflammation that develops within hours and can last 2–3 days. Prevalence of this event may reach 25 % of patients and does not predict a poor response to therapy. It is thought that the cause of the flare may be the excipients of the pharmacological preparation rather than the steroid itself.

Other events, such as subcutaneous fat atrophy, skin depigmentation, and tendon rupture, may be the consequence of incorrect injection technique. As far as steroids are injected in the correct location, the risk of such events is minimal. However, note that in particular procedures (e.g., when larger needles are used), steroids may reflux along needle track and producing the abovementioned complications. We suggest local compression (manually or with bandages) after steroid injection to avoid drug reflux.

Systemic effects occur following soft tissue or intra-articular injections but are generally believed to have minimal clinical importance. Nevertheless, it is important for the treating radiologist to be aware that intra-articular corticosteroids do exert variable systemic effects. Patients with diabetes who are administered such injections should thus be warned to expect a slight increase in their blood glucose level. In these patients, accurate blood glucose monitoring is recommended. Also, note that these patients are usually more prone to develop local infection; thus, higher caution should be taken.

Hyaluronic Acid

Intra-articular administration of hyaluronic acid, referred to as viscosupplementation, has been reported to be effective in the treatment of mild and moderate osteoarthritis. The aim of the procedure is to provide lubrication to the affected joint and to stimulate the production on endogenous synovial fluid, thus improving articular function.

Hyaluronic acid is long polymer composed by several molecules of N-acetylglucosamine and glucuronic acid linked together by glycosidic bonds. Hyaluronic acid is one of the main components of the extracellular matrix and can be found in the cartilage, synovial tissue, and synovial fluid. Hyaluronic acid has both mechanic (viscosupplementant) and pharmacologic (viscoinducent) properties, as it acts both as lubricant and shock absorbent and as promoter of endogenous synovial fluid.

Hyaluronic acid can be classified according to the weight of the polymer (low, intermediate, high molecular weight) and to the bindings that are present between them (no bindings, cross-linking, etc.). Acids with different molecular weight have different properties. The lower the molecular weight, the lower the mechanical properties, the higher the pharmacological action. Conversely, the higher the molecular weight, the higher the mechanical properties, the lower the pharmacological action. Cross-linkage can be also present in hyaluronic acids with higher molecular weight that further contribute in increasing the mechanical features. Persistence within joint space is also influenced by molecular weight. Low-weight hyaluronic acids have been reported to remain into joints for up to 4 days, while heavier acids have been reported to persist up to 4 weeks.

Platelet-Rich Plasma

Platelet-rich plasma (PRP) is derived from three components (platelet concentrate, cryoprecipitate of fibrinogen, and thrombin) that are withdrawn from fresh blood of the patient and combined together prior to injection. After blood withdrawal, PRP can be prepared by hematology service of the hospital or using commercial kits. Once activated with 1–2 ml of 10 % calcium gluconate, PRP should be injected immediately to avoid gelification.

PRP is basically a platelet concentrate. Platelets contain several growth factors that contribute to promote healing of damaged tissues, in particular transforming growth factor-b (TGF-b), platelet-derived growth factor (PDGF), fibroblastic growth factor (FGF), and insulin-like growth factor (IGF). As degenerative tendinopathies are typically poorly vascularized, the use of PRP is thought to promote tendon healing.

The role of PRP in several branches of medicine, such as dentistry and maxillofacial and orthopedic surgery, is relatively consolidated. Regarding sport medicine, controversial results have been reported regarding the ability of PRP in promoting tendon healing more efficiently than simple needling or other less invasive, expensive treatments.

Post-procedural Care

Generally speaking, after superficial interventional procedures, the needle access is covered with a simple plaster and/or relatively compressive bandage. The patient may also benefit of ice pack positioned over the treated joint. For more invasive procedures, we suggest to monitor the patient for 15–30 min after treatment, to take care of possible adverse events that may occur. Also, oral administration of a short course of anti-inflammatory drugs and/or painkillers may be advisable in some cases. We do not routinely administer antibiotic therapy in patients undergoing US-guided interventional procedures of the musculoskeletal system; however, particular patients (e.g., diabetic patients) may require extra caution. Last, patients should be instructed on how to behave after the treatment (rest period, physiokinesis therapy, etc.) and possibly given a contact (telephone number, e-mail address) to contact in case of unexpected events (Figs. 1.2 and 1.3).

Acknowledgement This chapter is partially based on Chapter 1 of the volume *Ultrasound-guided Musculoskeletal Procedures. The Upper Limb*. The authors wish to acknowledge the collaboration of Armando Conchiglia, Lorenzo Maria Gregori, Luigi Zugaro, and Carlo Masciocchi.

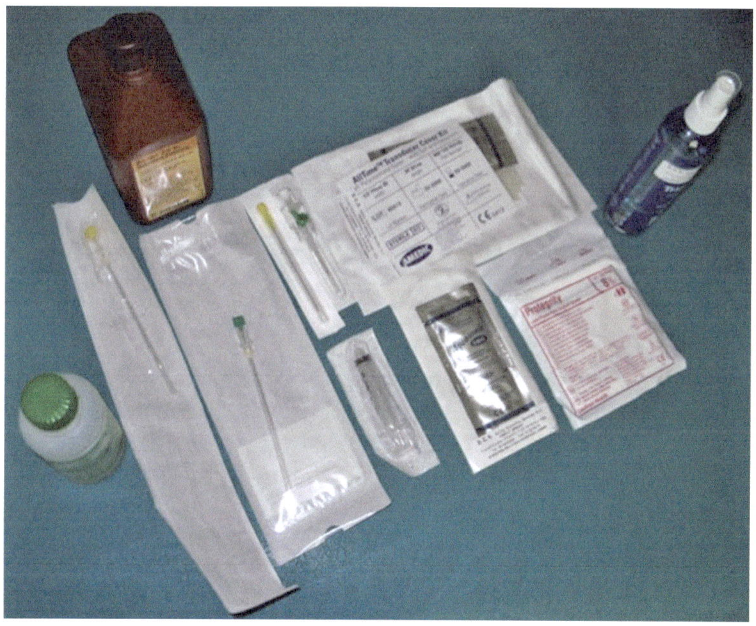

Fig. 1.2 Material required to perform US-guided musculoskeletal procedures: syringes, antiseptic solutions, needles, sterile probe cover, sterile gel, and gloves

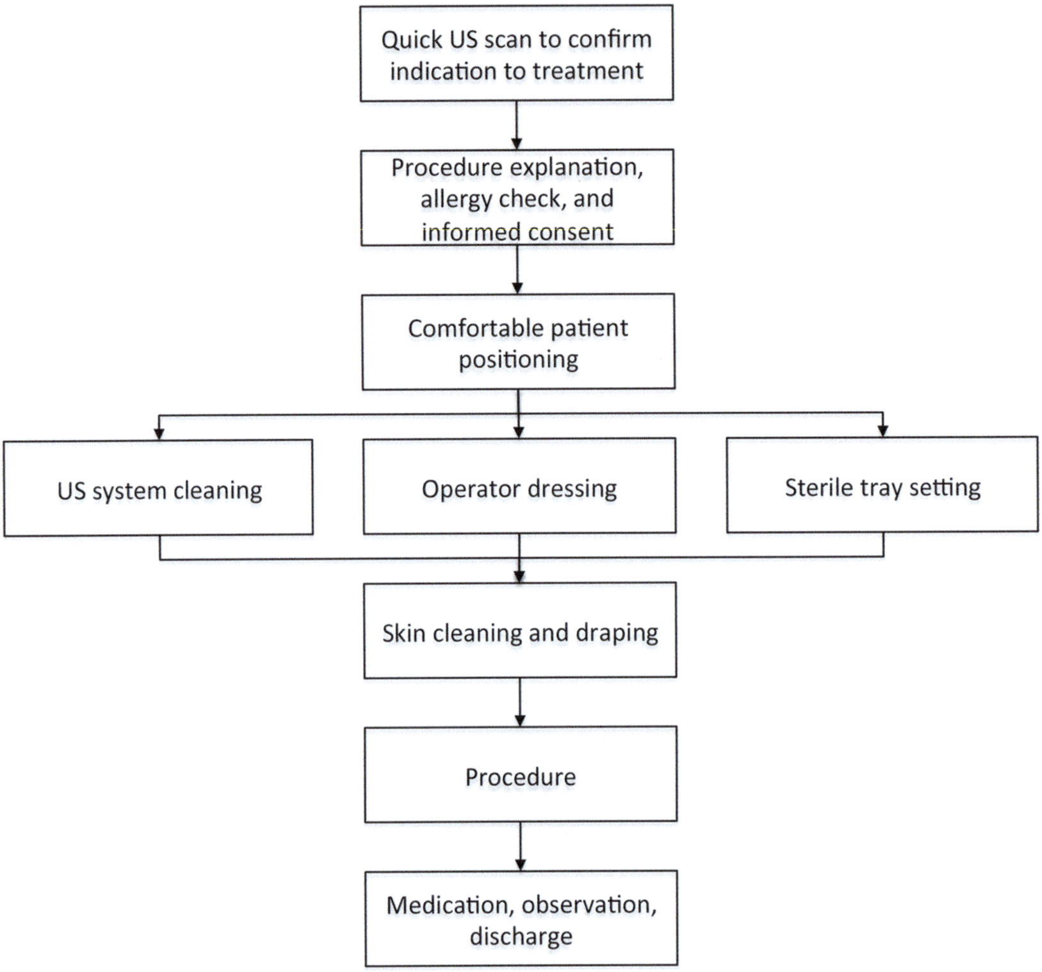

Fig. 1.3 General workflow for US-guided interventional procedures

Part I

The Hip

2 The Hip: Focused Ultrasound Anatomy and Examination Technique

Emanuele Fabbro and Giulio Ferrero

Focused Ultrasound Anatomy and Examination Technique

The hip can be divided into four compartments: anterior, medial, lateral and posterior.

Anterior Compartment

Sartorius and Tensor Fasciae Latae

Anatomy

The sartorius and the tensor fasciae latae muscles are the superficial group of the anterior hip muscles, and they arise, respectively, from the medial and the lateral side of the anterior superior iliac spine (ASIS).

The sartorius muscle courses distally and obliquely, superficially to the deep group of thigh muscles, reaching the anteromedial aspect of the proximal leg; the tensor fasciae latae muscle courses distally on the lateral side of the thigh. The sartorius muscle ends at the pes anserinus, that is, the conjoined insertion of three tendons (sartorius, gracilis, semitendinosus) onto the anteromedial surface of the proximal extremity of the tibia; the tensor fasciae latae muscle inserts through the iliotibial band onto the Gerdy's tubercle, located at the anterolateral aspect of the proximal tibial epiphysis.

Scanning Technique

The patient lies supine on the table with the lower limb extended in a neutral position. After having found the ASIS with palpation, the probe is placed on it in a horizontal position to visualise the typical "pseudo-thyroid" aspect with the hyperechoic ASIS at the centre, next to the short tendinous insertions of the sartorius (medial) and the tensor fasciae latae (lateral) muscles. Gliding caudally, the muscle bellies are examined using both axial and longitudinal scans (Fig. 2.1).

E. Fabbro (✉) • G. Ferrero
Unit of Radiology, Ospedale Santa Corona,
ASL 2 Savonese, Pietra Ligure, Italy
e-mail: emanuele.fabbro@gmail.com;
giulio.ferrero@gmail.com

L.M. Sconfienza et al. (eds.), *Ultrasound-guided Musculoskeletal Procedures: The Lower Limb*, DOI 10.1007/978-88-470-5764-7_2

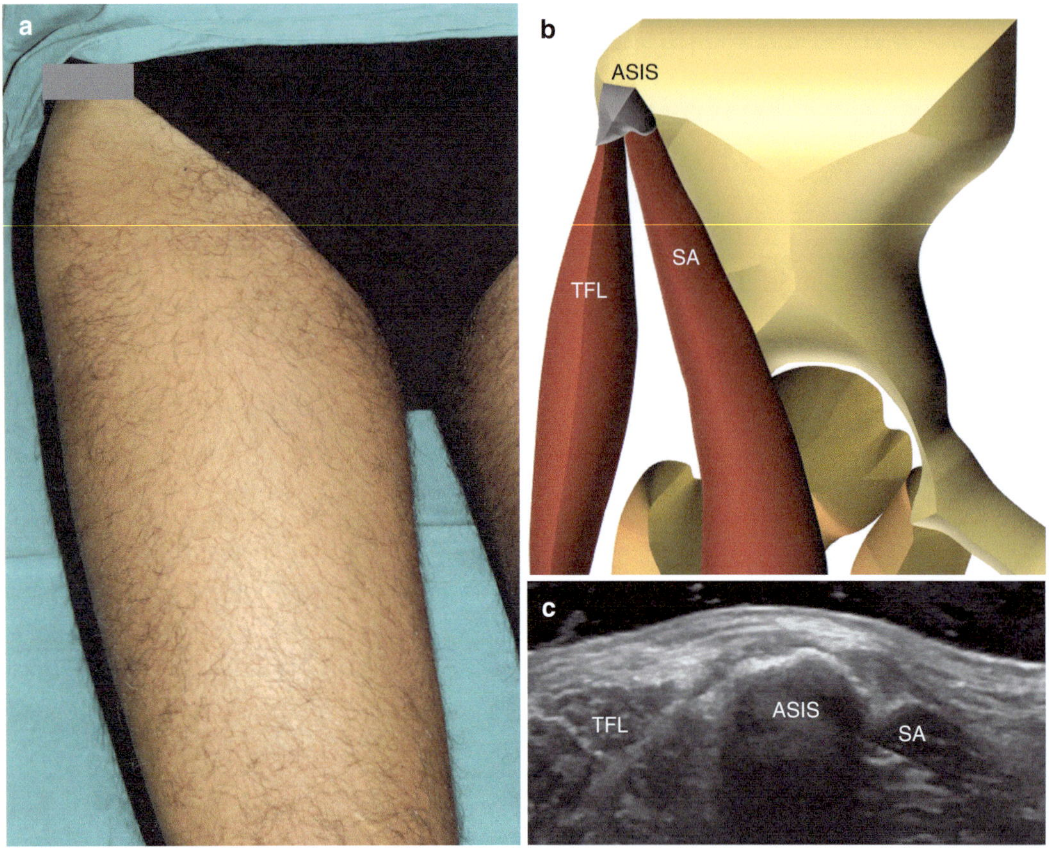

Fig. 2.1 Evaluation of the anterior superior iliac spine to assess the tensor fasciae latae and the sartorius tendons and muscles. (**a**) The probe and patient are positioned to evaluate the anterior superior iliac spine on a short-axis scan. (**b**) Anatomical scheme of the anterior superior iliac spine and the tensor fasciae latae and the sartorius tendons and muscles as seen along their short axis. *TFL* tensor fasciae latae, *ASIS* anterior superior iliac spine, *SA* sartorius. (**c**) US short-axis scan of the anterior superior iliac spine, the tensor fasciae latae and the sartorius tendons and muscles

Rectus Femoris and Iliopsoas Muscles

Anatomy

The rectus femoris muscle is part of the deep group of the anterior compartment muscles of the hip, and it belongs to the quadriceps femoris complex. It inserts over the anterior inferior iliac spine (AIIS) with three different proximal tendons: the direct tendon, inserting directly on the AIIS; the indirect tendon, which is an aponeurosis into the muscle belly, running under the direct tendon proximally and then coursing externally; and the reflected tendon that anchors the chondrolabral complex of the hip joint. The rectus femoris muscle crosses the anterior aspect of the hip, coursing the anterior thigh to insert into the upper pole of the patella through the quadriceps tendon.

The iliopsoas muscle is composed of two muscles arising from the posterior abdominal wall: the psoas major and the iliacus. The psoas muscle arises from the transverse processes and the body of T12–L5 vertebrae and the lateral aspects of the discs between them; the iliacus muscle originates from the iliac fossa. The muscle belly runs obliquely down and outwards, it passes under the inguinal ligament and it inserts onto the apex of the lesser trochanter through a common tendon.

Between the joint capsule and the posterior surface of the iliopsoas muscle, there is the iliopsoas bursa, the largest synovial bursa of the human body, which communicates with the joint space in 15 % of cases.

Scanning Technique

Starting with the probe at ASIS level in horizontal position, the transducer is shifted caudally to reach the AIIS and to visualise the direct tendon of the rectus femoris muscle in its axial scan, lateral to the iliopsoas muscle. The direct and indirect tendons of the rectus femoris can be evaluated using axial and longitudinal scans. From this position, the transducer is shifted caudally to reach the muscle belly of the rectus femoris; then the probe can be rotated 90° clockwise to evaluate, by longitudinal scans, the myotendinous junctions of the rectus up to the insertion onto the AIIS.

To evaluate the iliopsoas, the probe is placed slightly medially to the AIIS, and a series of axial scans are used to detect the iliopsoas muscle. The muscle can be followed using both axial and longitudinal scans up to the insertion onto the lesser trochanter (Fig. 2.2).

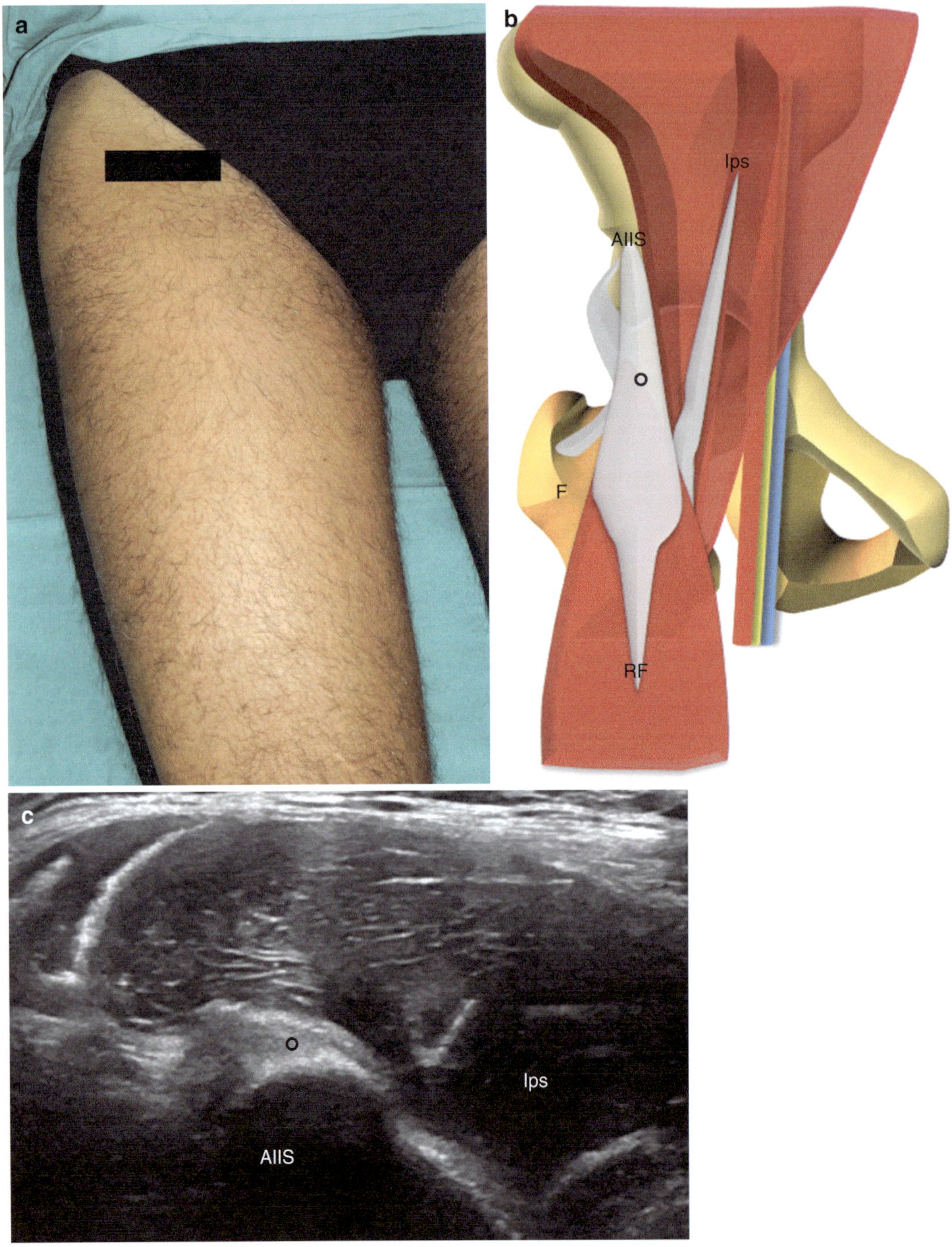

Fig. 2.2 Evaluation of the anterior thigh to assess the rectus femoris and the iliopsoas. (**a**) The probe and patient are positioned to evaluate the rectus femoris and the iliopsoas on a short-axis scan. (**b**) Anatomical scheme of the rectus femoris and the iliopsoas as seen along their short axis. *AIIS* anterior inferior iliac spine, *circle* rectus femoris conjoined tendon, *RF* rectus femoris muscle, *Ips* iliopsoas muscle, *F* femur. (**c**) US short-axis scan of the rectus femoris and the iliopsoas. The iliopsoas bursa is not visible in normal conditions

Hip Joint

Anatomy

The hip is a joint composed by the acetabulum and the femoral neck. It is a deep joint, covered by thick muscles, namely, the quadriceps and the iliopsoas. Using US, only the most superficial structures can be seen, namely, the femoral head with its articular cartilage, the anterior lateral border of acetabulum, the anterior lateral labrum and the anterior joint capsule. The intra-articular space cannot be evaluated using US.

Scanning Technique

The probe should be placed slightly medially and distally to the AIIS. Orientation of the probe could be purely sagittal – to visualise the joint space or sagittal oblique – to localise the femoral head covered by the articular cartilage, the acetabulum, the anterior acetabular labrum, the head-neck junction and the hyperechoic anterior capsular profile. The anterior synovial recess, at the bottom of the femoral head, is not detectable when normal.

The anterior face of the femoral anatomical neck is intracapsular, covered by the joint capsule inserting into the acetabulum and the acetabular labrum, whereas the posterior side is only partially intracapsular, because of the joint capsule insertion between the medium and lateral third of the femoral neck (Fig. 2.3).

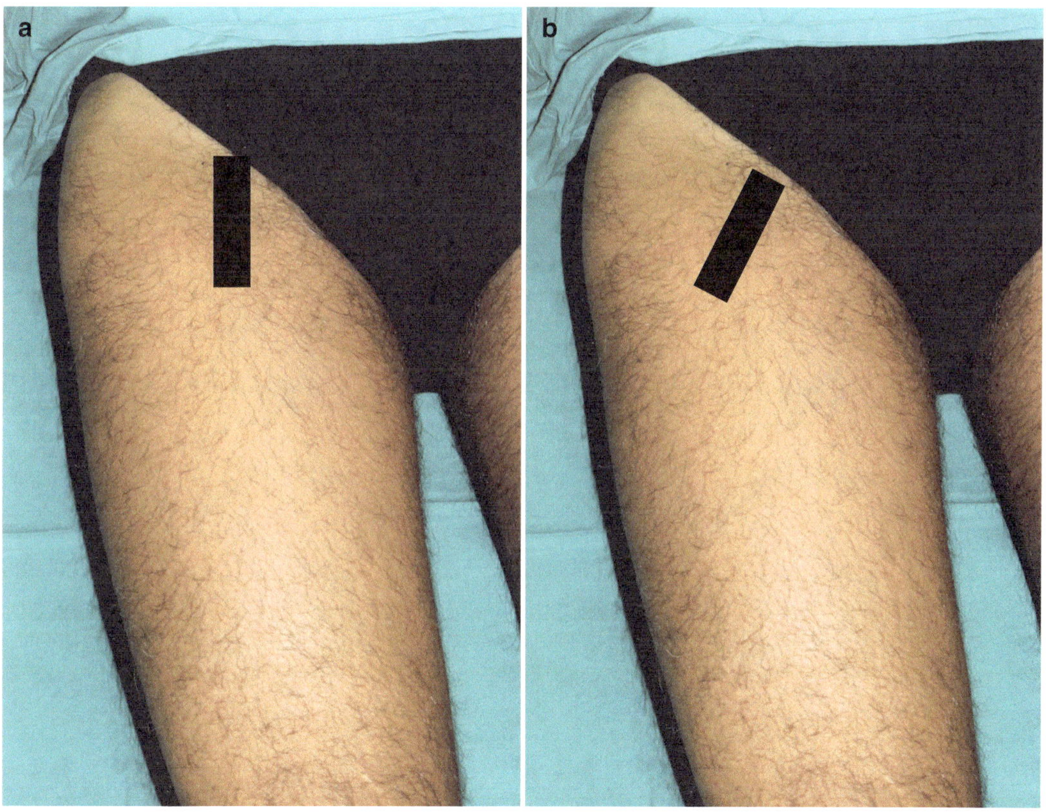

Fig. 2.3 Evaluation of the hip joint. (**a**, **b**) The probe and patient are positioned to evaluate the hip joint on sagittal and sagittal oblique scan, respectively. (**c**) Anatomical scheme of the hip joint. *A* acetabulum, *asterisk* labrum, *F* femoral head, *arrowheads* joint capsule, *Ps* iliopsoas muscle. (**d**, **e**) US scan of the hip joint on sagittal and sagittal oblique scan, respectively

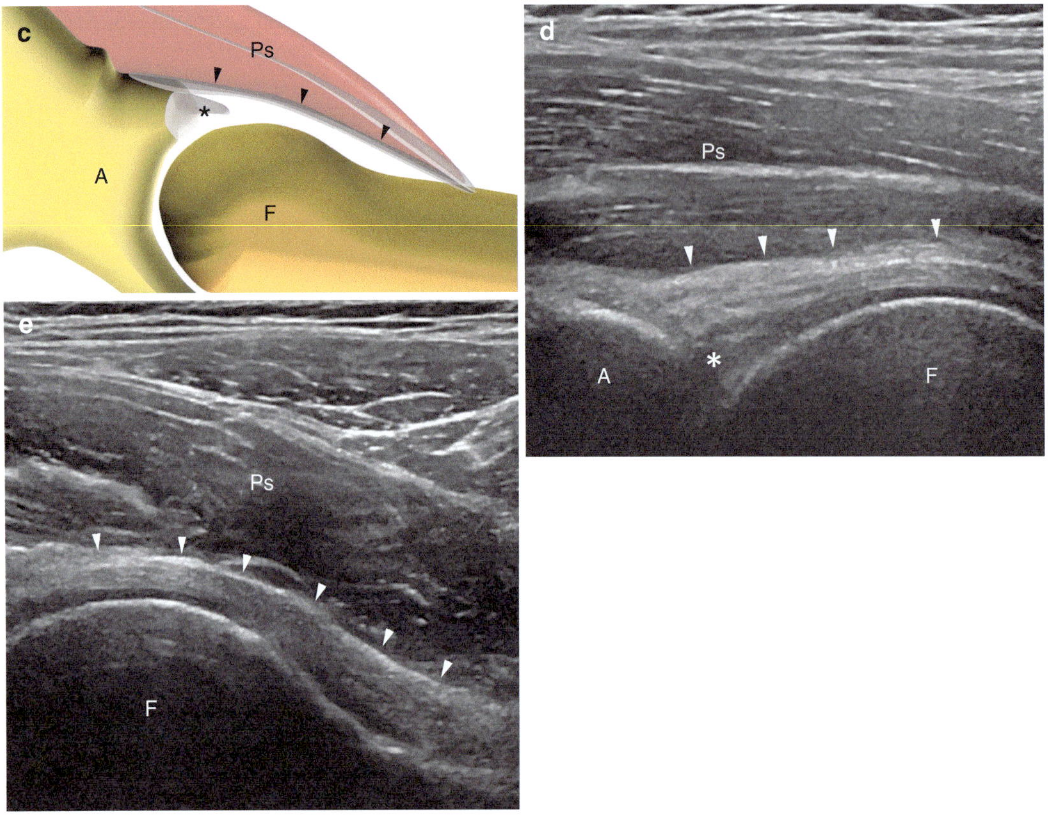

Fig. 2.3 (continued)

Medial Compartment

Adductor Tendons and Muscles

Anatomy

From the most superficial to the deepest layer, the adductor muscles include the adductor longus, the adductor brevis, the adductor magnus and the gracilis.

The adductor longus lies superficially and it arises from the body of the pubis, just inferior to the pubic crest. The adductor brevis originates from the inferior branch of the pubis. The adductor magnus, the largest of the adductors, arises from the inferior branch of the pubis, the ramus of the ischium and the ischial tuberosity. The gracilis is the most medial of the adductors, and it arises from the body and the inferior branch of the pubis. The first three muscles insert onto the femur, whereas the gracilis muscle ends at the pes anserinus.

Scanning Technique

The patient is supine, with the lower limb slightly externally rotated.

Placing the transducer in a longitudinal scan, the bony landmark of the pubic symphysis is identified to detect the adductor muscle tendon insertion. The probe is turned to detect each single muscle belly in both axial and longitudinal planes (Fig. 2.4).

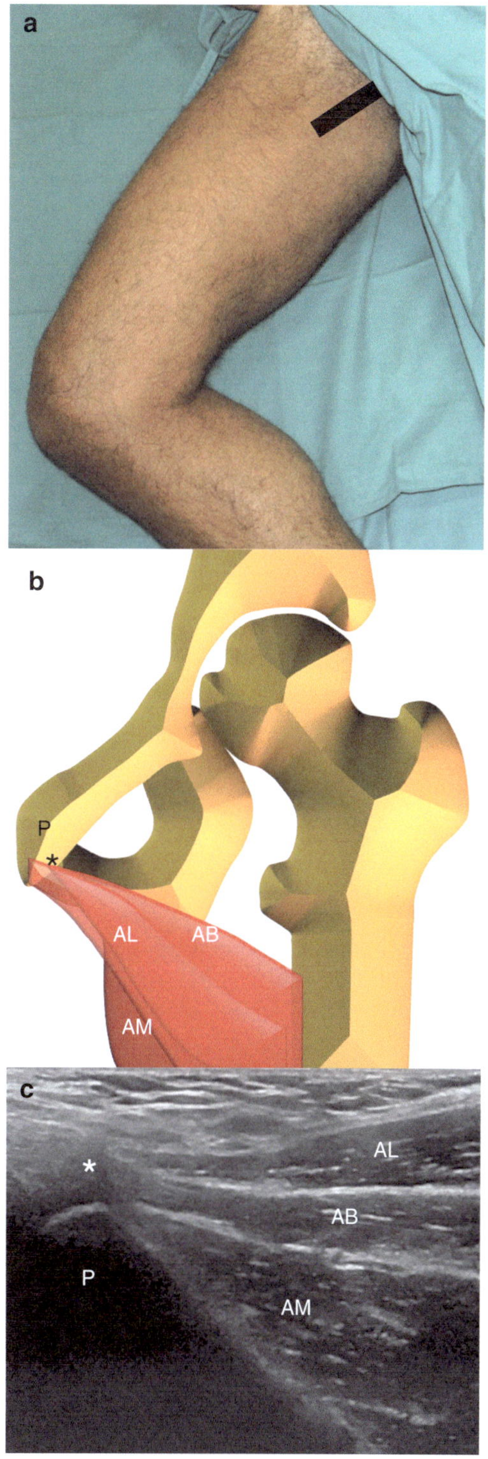

Fig. 2.4 Evaluation of the medial thigh to assess the adductor muscles. (**a**) The probe and patient are positioned to evaluate the adductor muscles on a long-axis scan. (**b**) Anatomical scheme of adductor muscles as seen along their long axis. *P* pubis, *asterisk* common adductor tendon, *AL* adductor longus muscle, *AB* adductor brevis muscle, *AM* adductor magnus muscle. (**c**) US long-axis scan of the adductor muscles

Lateral Compartment

Gluteus Tendons and Muscles

Anatomy

The muscles of the lateral compartment include essentially the gluteus medius and the gluteus minimus.

They originate from the posterior iliac wing. The gluteus minimus tendon inserts into the anterior facet of the greater trochanter. The anterior and middle portions of the gluteus medius insert into the lateral facet of the trochanter, whereas its posterior portion inserts into the posterosuperior facet of the greater trochanter.

There are two trochanteric bursae: the trochanteric bursa of the gluteus medius that separates its tendon from the anterosuperior side of the greater trochanter and the trochanteric bursa of the gluteus maximus, often multilocular, that separates the deep side of the gluteus maximus from the posterolateral bony surface of the greater trochanter.

Superficially to glutei muscles, the tendinous portion of the tensor fasciae latae can be visualised as a hyperechoic structure separated from the abductor tendon cuff of the hip by the synovial bursa and adipose cleavage planes.

Scanning Technique

The patient lies in a lateral position, on the contralateral hip.

The probe is placed horizontally to find the greater trochanter and then it is shifted slightly cranially. Gliding the transducer from posterior to anterior, the muscles of the lateral compartment can be identified (Fig. 2.5).

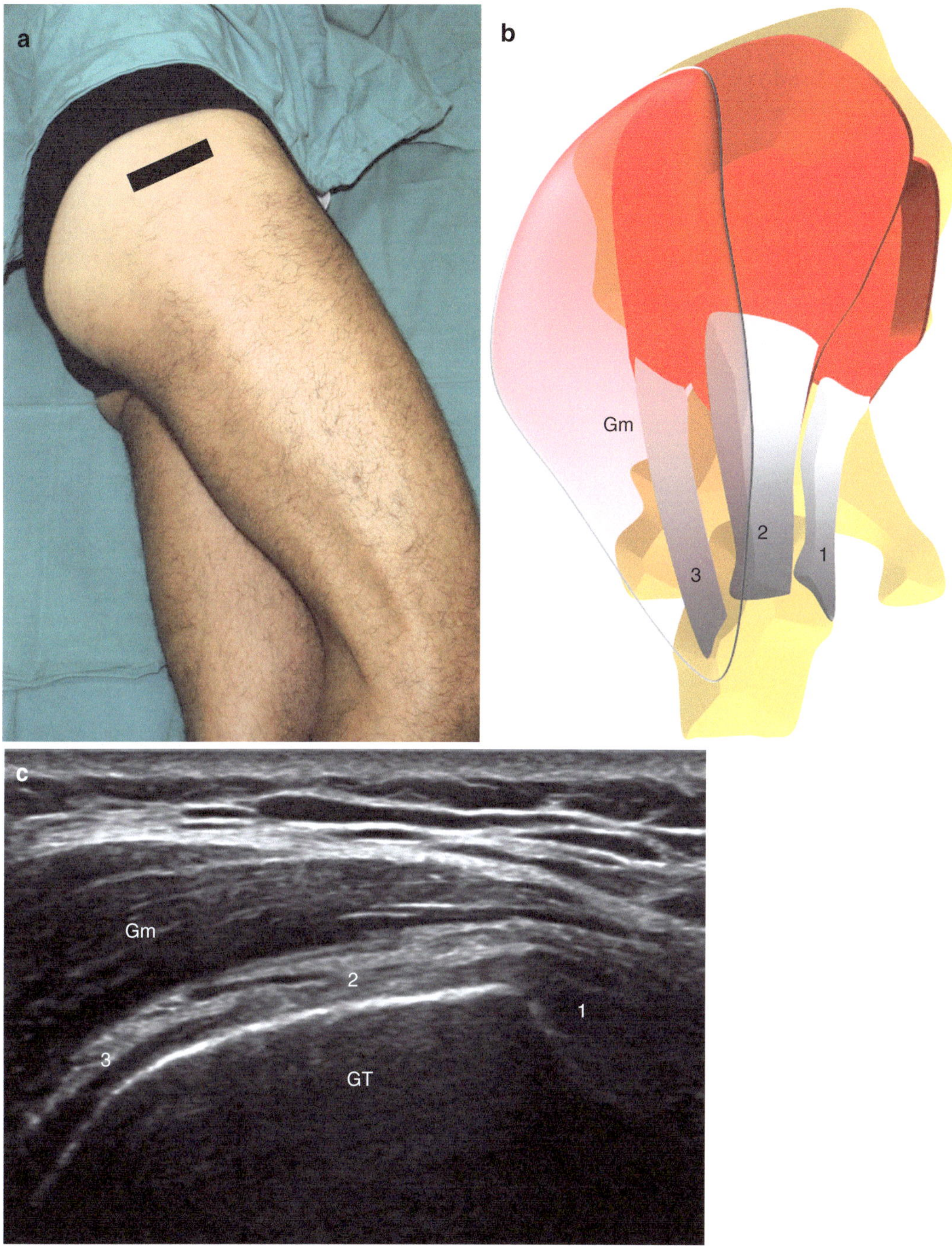

Fig. 2.5 Evaluation of the lateral thigh to assess the gluteal tendons and muscles. (**a**) The probe and patient are positioned to evaluate the gluteal tendons and muscles on a short-axis scan. (**b**) Anatomical scheme of the gluteal tendons and muscles as seen along their short axis. *GT* greater trochanter; *1* tendon of gluteus minimus; *2* and *3* anterior and posterior tendons, respectively, of gluteus medius; *Gm* gluteus maximus muscle. (**c**) US short-axis scan of the gluteal tendons and muscles

Posterior Compartment

Ischiocrural Tendons (Hamstrings) and Sciatic Nerve

Anatomy

The deep layer of posterior hip muscles consists of three ischiocrural muscles: the long head of the biceps femoris, the semitendinosus and the semimembranosus.

These muscles arise from the ischiatic tuberosity and course inferiorly to insert into the leg. The long head of biceps femoris and the semitendinosus have a conjoined tendon which originates from the lateral aspect of the ischiatic tuberosity. The semimembranosus tendon arises more medially, from the inferior aspect of the ischiatic tuberosity.

Scanning Technique

The patient lies prone with the lower limb in a neutral position. The probe is placed horizontally to find the ischiatic tuberosity and to visualise the proximal tendon insertion of the ischiocrural muscles on it. From lateral to medial, the long head of the biceps femoris, the semitendinosus and the semimembranosus tendons are seen. Lateral to the hamstrings' insertion, the sciatic nerve can also be seen (Fig. 2.6).

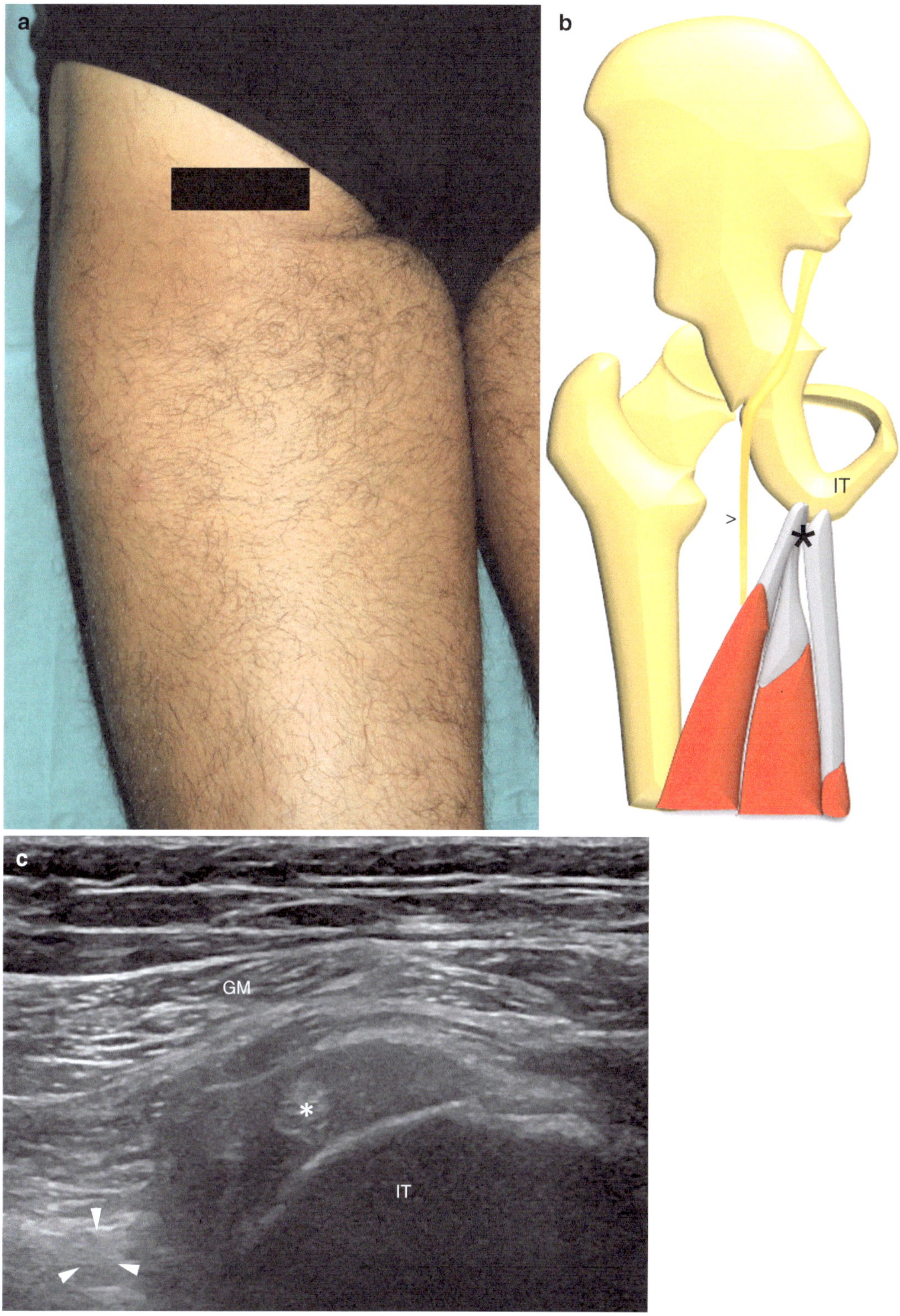

Fig. 2.6 Evaluation of the posterior thigh to assess the insertion of the hamstring tendons. (**a**) The probe and patient are positioned to evaluate the hamstring tendons on a short-axis scan. (**b**) Anatomical scheme of the hamstring tendons as seen along their short axis. *IT* ischiatic tuberosity, *asterisk* insertion of the hamstring tendons, *arrowheads* sciatic nerve, *GM* gluteus maximus muscle. (**c**) US short-axis scan of the hamstring tendons

3 Hip Intra-articular Injections

Emanuele Fabbro and Giulio Ferrero

Essentials

Intra-articular injections of the hip can be performed to treat a number of pathologic conditions. The drugs administered in these cases may be anti-inflammatory agents, such as steroids that may be indicated for patients with advanced hip osteoarthritis (OA) refractory to other treatments or viscosupplementants, such as hyaluronic acid, that can be used to treat patients with mild to moderate OA. Anesthetics may be injected for diagnostic purposes to differentiate intra- and extra-articular pathology.

Hip OA

Hip OA is a very common condition and affects 4.4 % of adults over 55 years, with progressive increase with aging. Primary hip OA is a degenerative joint disease frequently associated with aging and increased loads on this weight-bearing joint, two conditions that frequently coexist. Secondary hip OA can be found in patients with untreated femoroacetabular impingement or hip dysplasia, in which altered biomechanics usually lead to joint damage.

E. Fabbro (✉) • G. Ferrero
Unit of Radiology, Ospedale Santa Corona,
ASL 2 Savonese, Pietra Ligure, Italy
e-mail: emanuele.fabbro@gmail.com;
giulio.ferrero@gmail.com

Clinical Presentation

The main symptom is joint stiffness that occurs as they are getting out of bed or after sitting for a long time, variably associated with pain, swelling, or tenderness in the hip joint and inability to move the hip to perform routine activities, such as exiting from the car or putting on socks. Sometimes, a sound or feeling of bone rubbing against bone is reported.

Ultrasound Diagnosis

The diagnosis of hip OA requires plain film examination. However, US can demonstrate the presence of joint effusion, thickened and/or calcified capsule, and calcifications of the acetabular labrum. Magnetic resonance imaging may be required to detect the presence of associated abnormalities.

Treatment Options

Conservative treatment includes weight loss, physical therapy, oral anti-inflammatory and analgesic medications, and intra-articular injections (hyaluronic acid, steroids). At later stage, total hip replacement can be performed.

L.M. Sconfienza et al. (eds.), *Ultrasound-guided Musculoskeletal Procedures: The Lower Limb*, DOI 10.1007/978-88-470-5764-7_3

Interventional Procedure

Indications

Differential diagnosis between extra- and intra-articular pathology: anesthetic injection

Painful primary or secondary OA, conservative treatment in patients ineligible for total hip arthroplasty: hyaluronic acid or steroid injection

Inflammatory arthritis: steroid injection

Intra-articular injections are generally contraindicated in patients with suspected or known joint infection, overlying cellulitis, or hypersensitivity to the pertinent drug.

This procedure can also be used to inject contrast agents within the joint for arthrography purposes.

Objective

To deliver anti-inflammatory, analgesic, or viscosupplementant drugs within the joint space

Equipment

- 1 syringe (2–5 ml)
- 20 G spinal needle
- Lidocaine 2 % (2–4 mL), long-acting steroid (1 ml, 40 mg/ml), or hyaluronic acid (2–6 ml)
- Plaster

How We Do It

Intra-articular injection at the level of the hip is generally more complex when compared to other joints (e.g., shoulder, knee) for its deep location and the relative contiguity of the femoral neurovascular bundle.

Lateral (in-plane) approach allows a direct and continuous visualization of the needle along the whole path in soft tissues, while out-plane approach may be preferred for being shorter and less painful, but needle visibility is remarkably decreased.

The patient lies in supine position. Slight internal rotation of the leg (about 15°–20°) may help to decrease joint capsule tension and improving tolerability of the procedure. The neurovascular bundle can be visualized with an axial scan at the level of the groin to detect possible vascular or neural anatomic variations and avoid accidental punctures. Then, the probe is rotated about 135° and shifted laterally in order to reach an anterior sagittal-oblique scanning plane over the hip joint. A correct scanning plane should visualize the femoral neck, the femoral head covered by hyaline cartilage, the acetabular labrum, the osseous component of the acetabulum, the joint capsule, and, superficially, the iliopsoas muscle belly. The articular cortex of the femoral head appears as a curve echogenic line and the cortical surface of the anterior acetabular rim as a triangular echogenic structure just distal to this line. The fibrocartilaginous anterior acetabular labrum may be seen as a well-defined, triangular, and uniformly echogenic structure. Of note, in patients with advanced OA, anatomy of this joint can be relatively different, and joint components may be not identified easily.

Caudo-Cranial Approach

With the articular joint space centered in the middle of the screen, a 20 G spinal needle is inserted laterally to the distal side of the probe with a caudal-cranial direction. According to the patient's habitus, the depth of the joint may vary, and thus the angle of needle insertion has to be adjusted; generally, the angle of needle insertion ranges from 30° to 60°. Less experienced operators may take advantage of a metallic needle guide that can be attached to the ultrasound probe. With this approach, the whole path of the needle can be visualized in real time, and slight corrections of the direction can be made. The needle tip can be inserted in within the whole joint capsule. However, inserting the needle exactly in the joint space may result in a very painful injection procedure. The best area to put the needle tip is at the femoral head-neck junction. Once the joint space is reached, the syringe is connected to the needle, and the drug is injected. Of note, in case of high resistance to injection, the needle should be minimally retracted.

This procedure can be also performed with the cranial-caudal approach. Power Doppler module can also be switched on to monitor the flow of the drug within the capsule during injection.

At the end of the injection, the needle can be removed and a plaster should be applied.

The procedure is shown in Fig. 3.1.

Coaxial Approach

The articular joint space is centered on the screen, and a 20 G spinal needle is inserted at the center of the longer side of the probe, with a very slight lateral-to-medial angulation (about 5°) to reach the joint space visualized in the scanning plane. Along its path, the needle tip is visualized indirectly, by means of slight movements of superficial soft tissues; when the joint space is reached, the needle tip should be visible as a hyperechoic dot under the articular capsule. Of note, this procedure is less painful for patients but requires longer experience in US-guided procedures.

Post-procedural Care

The patient is usually kept under observation for about 15 min after the procedure. Pain may occur after treatment and can be managed with a short course of oral NSAIDs.

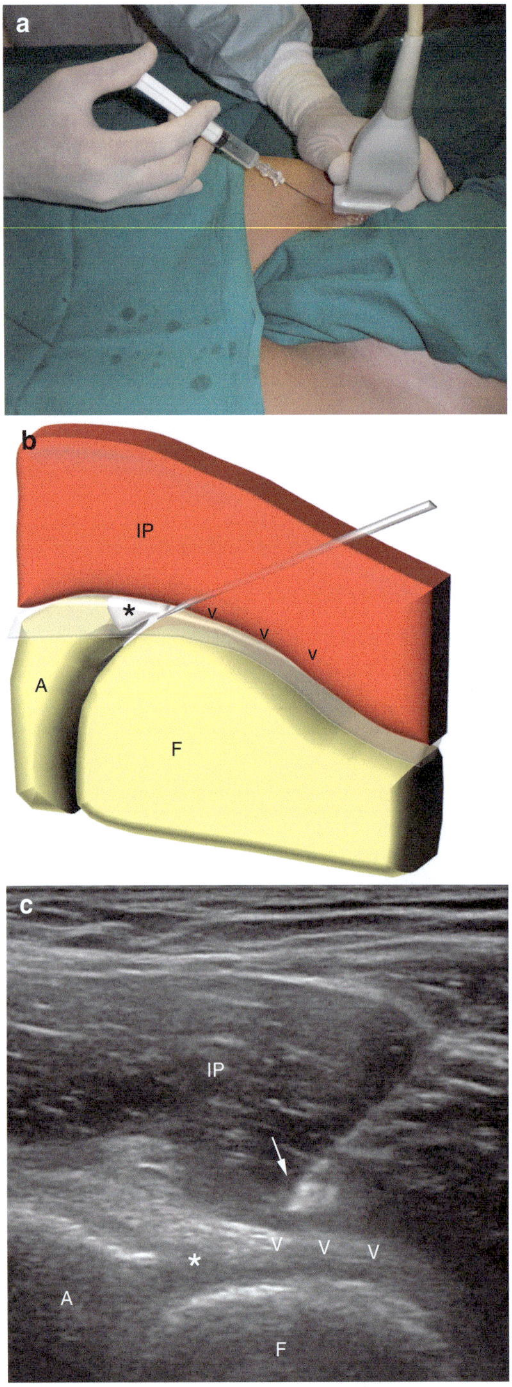

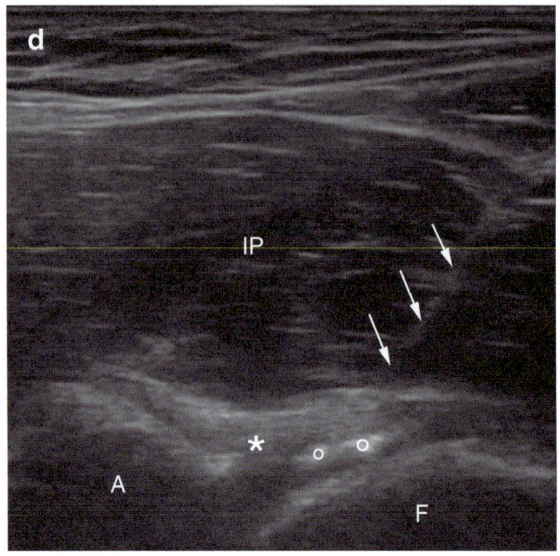

Fig. 3.1 US-guided intra-articular hip injection on a long-axis scan. (**a**) Probe and patient position to perform long-axis US-guided intra-articular hip injection. (**b**) Anatomical scheme and (**c**) US scan of long-axis intra-articular hip injection. *IP* iliopsoas muscle, *A* acetabulum, *F* femur, *asterisk* labrum, *arrow* needle tip, *arrowheads* joint capsule. (**d**) US scan showing hyaluronic acid (*circles*) intra-articular injection

4 Hip Insertional Tendinopathy

Giulio Ferrero, Emanuele Fabbro, and Angelo Corazza

Essentials

Tendons around the hip can develop degenerative changes at the site of insertion as a result of chronic microtraumatism due to overload or previous poorly healed acute injuries. Accurate anamnestic data collection and clinical examination are essential to differentiate this condition from acute or subacute traumatic injuries and other periarticular or intra-articular pathologies. Tendon insertions in the anteromedial and posterior compartments such as adductors, rectus femoris, and hamstrings are more frequently affected in young active individuals playing different sports like running, cycling, or football. On the other hand, chronic tendinopathy of the lateral compartment is most commonly found in middle-aged to elderly women and is generally referred to as "greater trochanteric pain syndrome" since it cannot be distinguished clinically from trochanteric bursitis, which the condition is often associated.

G. Ferrero (✉) • E. Fabbro
Unit of Radiology, Ospedale Santa Corona, ASL 2 Savonese, Pietra Ligure, Italy
e-mail: giulio.ferrero@gmail.com; emanuele.fabbro@gmail.com

A. Corazza
Postgraduate school in radiodiagnostics, University of Genova, School of Medicine, Genoa, Italy
e-mail: angelcoraz@libero.it

Clinical Presentation

The most common symptom is pain at the corresponding site of affected tendinous insertion, worsened by the execution of active movements against resistance, digital compression, or when lying on the affected side, without limitations in the hip range of motion. Attention must be paid to exclude abdominal causes of pain that can mimic adductor or rectus femoris tendinopathy. Hamstring enthesopathy can also mimic radiculopathy or be associated with sciatic nerve irritation.

Ultrasound Diagnosis

Ultrasound may help to place an accurate diagnosis. Degenerative tendinopathy may present with variable degree of tendon swelling and loss of fibrillar tendinous echotexture. Tiny hyperechoic calcifications at the site of insertion can also be seen. Of note, presence of symptoms is very important, as similar pathologic changes could often be found also in the contralateral tendon but remain asymptomatic. In more advanced cases, partial- or full-thickness tendon tears can be seen as focal anechoic areas with loss of normal fibrillar pattern. When present (e.g., iliopsoas, trochanter, etc.), a thickened, fluid-filled bursa can also be detected.

L.M. Sconfienza et al. (eds.), *Ultrasound-guided Musculoskeletal Procedures: The Lower Limb*, DOI 10.1007/978-88-470-5764-7_4

Treatment Options

Conservative treatment includes rest, weight loss, physical therapy, ice, and anti-inflammatory and analgesic medications. Pelvic imbalance (e.g., leg-length discrepancy) should always be excluded or corrected. In unresponsive cases, percutaneous ultrasound-guided procedures or surgical tendinous debridement can be considered.

Interventional Procedure

Indications

Symptomatic enthesopathy in one or more tendons around the hip.

Objective

To cause local hyperemia and bleeding into the tendon, thus promoting post-procedural platelet-induced recovery phenomena.

Equipment

- 1 syringe (5–10 ml)
- 20 G spinal needle
- Lidocaine (5–10 ml)
- Long-acting steroid (1 ml, 40 mg/ml)
- Plaster

How We Do It

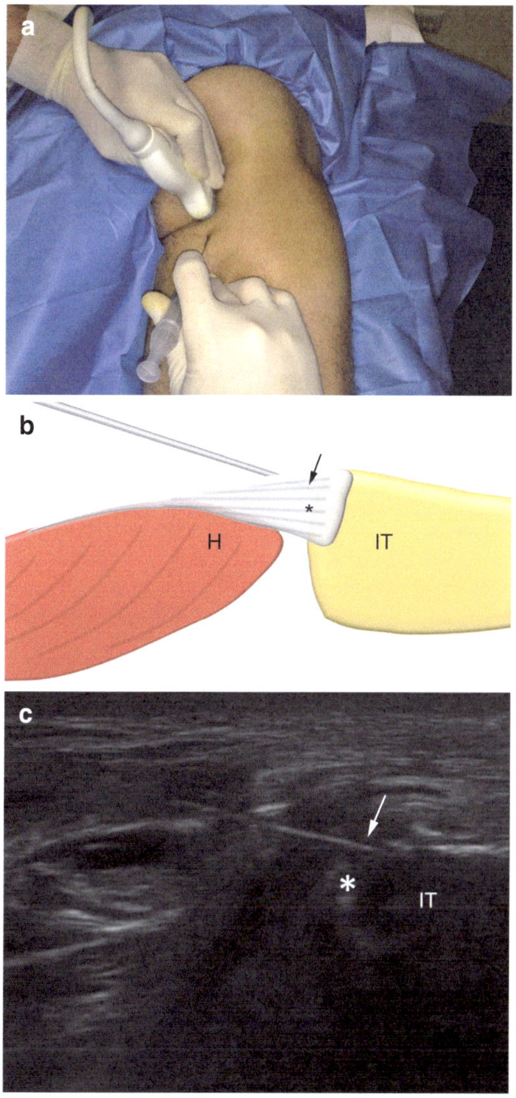

Fig. 4.1 US-guided treatment of hamstring tendinopathy on a long-axis scan. (**a**) Probe and patient position to perform long-axis US-guided treatment of hamstring tendinopathy. (**b**) Anatomical scheme and (**c**) US scan of hamstring tendinopathy treatment. *H* hamstring muscle, *asterisk* tendon slip, *IT* ischiatic tuberosity, *arrow* needle tip

STEP 1

The patient is positioned in a different way according to the tendon to treat (see below). A US scan is made to identify the insertional portion and to assess the most comfortable percutaneous approach. Whatever the chosen approach, the purpose is to position the needle tip within the affected area of the tendon.

Hamstring enthesopathy: the patient is positioned prone and tendinous insertions are demonstrated by means of a parasagittal US scan. Discrete pressure on the probe could be necessary according to patient's habitus. The needle is then inserted with an in-plane, caudal-to-cranial approach. The procedure is shown in **Fig. 4.1**.

Rectus femoris enthesopathy: the patient lies in supine position with the lower limb in neutral position. The proximal tendinous insertion is assessed by means of both transverse and longitudinal scans, and the needle is inserted with an in-plane medial-to-lateral or caudo-cranial approach. The procedure is shown in **Fig. 4.2**.

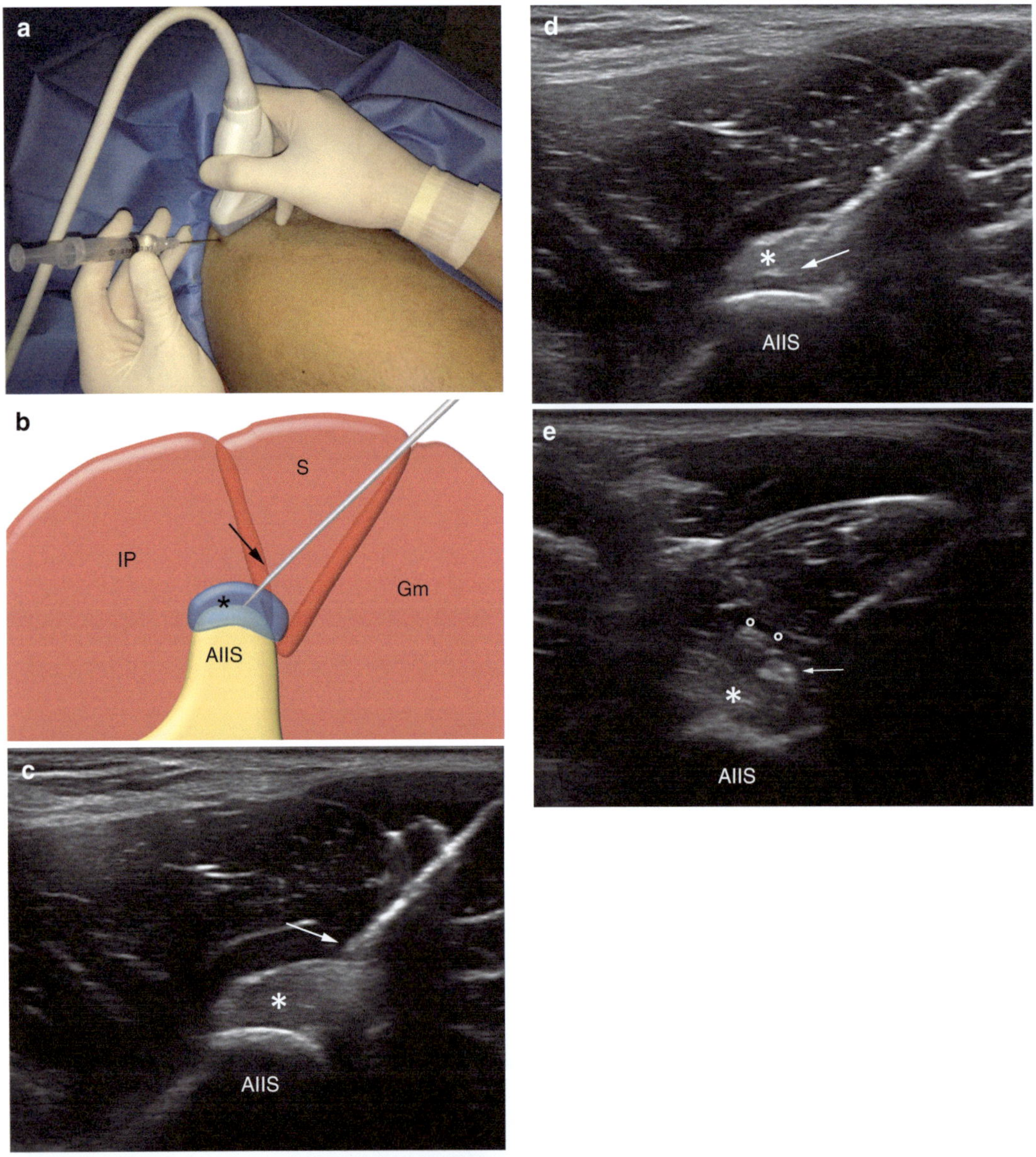

Fig. 4.2 US-guided treatment of rectus femoris tendinopathy on a short-axis scan. (**a**) Probe and patient position to perform short-axis US-guided treatment of rectus femoris tendinopathy. (**b**) Anatomical scheme and (**c**) US scan of rectus femoris tendinopathy treatment. *IP* iliopsoas muscle, *S* sartorius muscle, *Gm* gluteus maximus muscle, *asterisk* tendon slip, *AIIS* anterior inferior iliac spine, *arrow* needle tip. (**d**) Peritendinous anesthetic (*circles*) injection. (**e**) Dry-needling procedure

Trochanteric enthesopathy: the patient lies on the contralateral side. The affected tendon is demonstrated with an axial scan over the trochanter avoiding to apply excessive pressure to detect if trochanteric bursitis is associated. The needle is then inserted with a posterior-to-anterior, medial-to-lateral, in-plane approach. The procedure is shown in **Fig. 4.3**.

Adductors enthesopathy: the patient lies in supine position with the lower limb in slight extrarotation. The proximal tendinous insertion is assessed with a longitudinal scan, and the needle is inserted with an in-plane caudo-cranial approach.

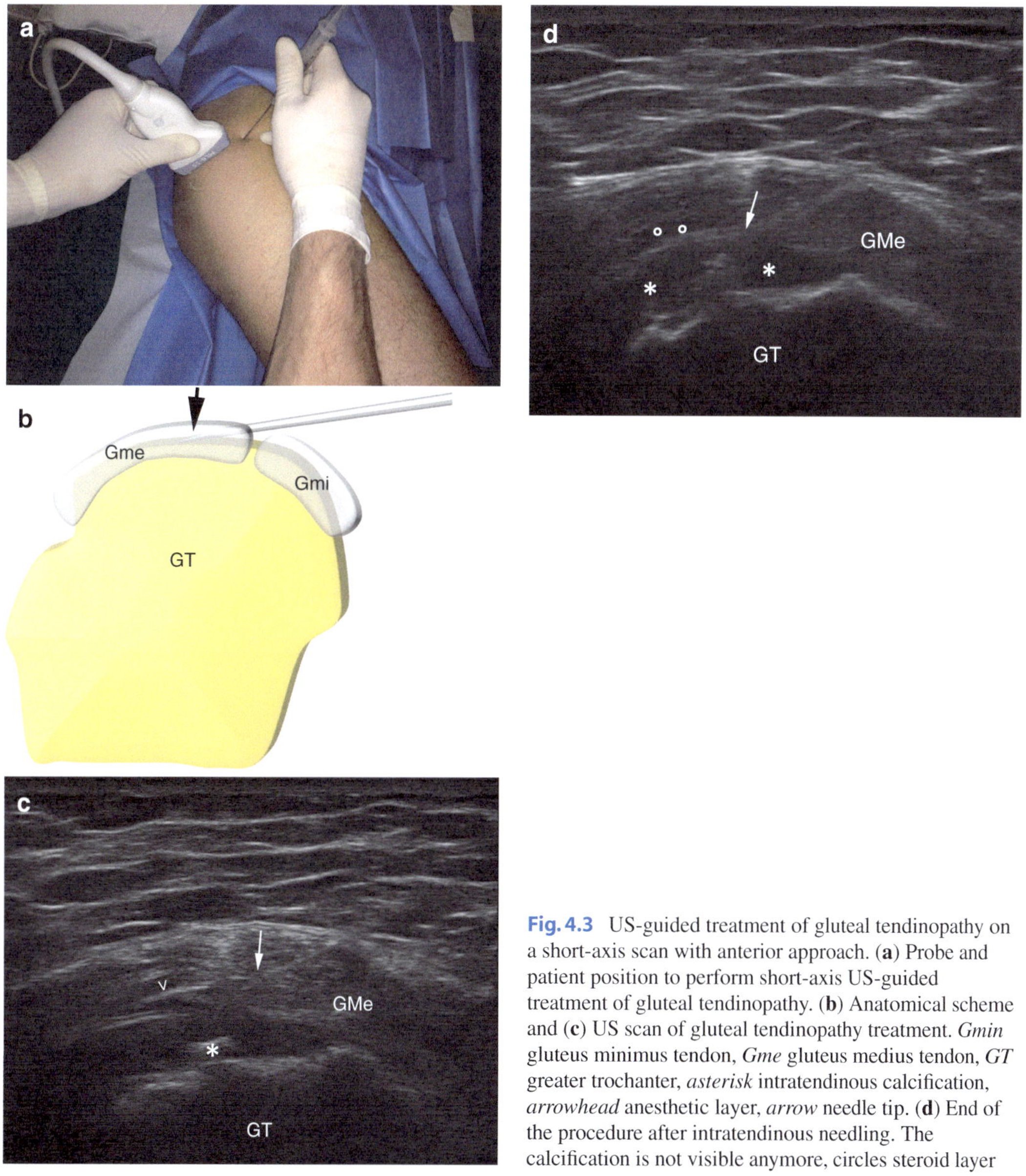

Fig. 4.3 US-guided treatment of gluteal tendinopathy on a short-axis scan with anterior approach. (**a**) Probe and patient position to perform short-axis US-guided treatment of gluteal tendinopathy. (**b**) Anatomical scheme and (**c**) US scan of gluteal tendinopathy treatment. *Gmin* gluteus minimus tendon, *Gme* gluteus medius tendon, *GT* greater trochanter, *asterisk* intratendinous calcification, *arrowhead* anesthetic layer, *arrow* needle tip. (**d**) End of the procedure after intratendinous needling. The calcification is not visible anymore, circles steroid layer

STEP 2

A small amount of anesthetic is injected around the area to treat. After a couple of minutes waiting without retracting the needle, a series of 15–20 repeated punctures (dry-needling) on the affected portion of the tendon is then performed. When the enthesis is affected, the periosteum should also be hit.

STEP 3

Half to one mL of steroid is injected in the peritendinous soft tissues, superficially to tendon enthesis. Caution should be taken to avoid direct intratendinous injection. When a bursa is present, the steroid should be preferably injected therein.

At the end of the procedure, the needle is then removed and a plaster applied at the cutaneous puncture site.

Post-procedure Care

The patient is kept in observation for about 10 min. A rest period of the affected structure and associated physical therapy are suggested. Pain after treatment may occur and it could be managed using ice and oral NSAIDs.

5 Periarticular Fluid Collections

Luca Maria Sconfienza and Alice Arcidiacono

Essentials

Despite the fact of being a weight-bearing joint, the hip is not really prone to develop large intra-articular effusion. When this happens, synovial fluid may be aspirated using the same procedure reported priorly to perform intra-articular injections. Conversely, periarticular fluid collections may be relatively more frequent.

In patients who underwent total hip replacement, periarticular fluid collections may involve the periarticular soft tissues and the overlying muscle, up to reaching the subcutaneous tissues and the skin. There, collection may create small sinus tracts or fistulae draining the collection content. These collections may be due to infection, bleeding, or inflammatory reaction and may contain pus, blood, or serum, respectively. In some cases, these collections turn out to be very dense (e.g., in case of chronic blood collections) or solid, forming periarticular masses that are called pseudotumors. They are mainly caused by a granulomatous adverse reaction to the implant itself.

Patients who suffered a direct trauma on the hip may develop subcutaneous sero-hematic fluid collections. This is particularly frequent in motorbikers that fall on the hip. These collections are named Morel-Lavallée lesions and are caused by the shear trauma that implies the detachment of the subcutaneous fat from the underlying muscular fascia.

Clinical Presentation

Clinical presentation may remarkably vary.

In patients with total hip replacement, the hip may be asymptomatic or give different degrees of discomfort. Usually, swelling may be seen or palpated over the anterior/lateral aspect of the hip. In case of infected collection, the skin and the surgical scar may be particularly red and temperature may be present. Blood test may reveal increase in white blood cell count and inflammatory indexes.

In patients who suffered a direct trauma, pain is usually present, together with swelling of the lateral aspect of the hip, especially over the greater trochanter. The overlying skin is usually normal.

L.M. Sconfienza (✉)
Unit of Radiology, IRCCS Policlinico San Donato, Milan, Italy

Department of Biomedical Sciences for Health, University of Milano, Milano, Italy
e-mail: io@lucasconfienza.it

A. Arcidiacono
Postgraduate school in Radiodiagnostics, University of Genova, School of Medicine, Genoa, Italy
e-mail: alice.arcidiacono@hotmail.com

L.M. Sconfienza et al. (eds.), *Ultrasound-guided Musculoskeletal Procedures: The Lower Limb*, DOI 10.1007/978-88-470-5764-7_5

Ultrasound Diagnosis

Ultrasound is particularly helpful to confirm the diagnosis of periarticular fluid collections, although small collections may be overlooked.

In patients with total hip replacement, ultrasound may demonstrate the presence of hypo-/anechoic area over the anterior/lateral aspect of the hip. Usually, abdominal convex transducer may help to evaluate the presence of deeper collections that involve the joint space.

In patients with a Morel-Lavallée lesion, ultrasound usually demonstrates the presence of an anechoic subcutaneous collection extending over the lateral aspect of the hip. Occasionally, some hyperechoic lobules can be detected within the collection, representing fat lobules of the subcutaneous fat layer.

In both cases, the use of the extended field of view (EFOV) module may help depicting the whole extension of the collection.

Treatment Options

In patients with total hip replacement, large fluid collections need to be drained to perform microbiological analysis. In patients with mass-like lesions, aspiration is usually not possible and biopsy with a Tru-Cut needle should be performed.

Patients with Morel-Lavallée lesions are usually treated conservatively with compression bandages until complete resolution. However, larger collections may not resolve spontaneously and may take advantage of percutaneous aspiration.

Interventional Procedure

Indications and Objective

Diagnostic and therapeutic aspiration and drainage of peri-prosthetic or subcutaneous fluid collections.

Equipment

- 1 syringe (20–50 ml)
- 14-16-18 G needle
- Biopsy handle
- Bandages
- Plaster

How We Do It

STEP 1

The patient is positioned in a different way according to the area to aspirate. Generally, however, the patient should be positioned on the contralateral hip to have full access to the anterior and the lateral aspect of the affected joint. A thorough US scan is made to identify the area to aspirate and to plan the best access path.

STEP 2

A large needle connected to a syringe is inserted with an in-plane approach until the needle tip enters the collection. Of note, larger needles are usually needed, as small needles tend to be obstructed by clots or by fat lobules. Occasionally, hematic content may be very dense and drainage could be challenging. In this case, the operator may inject in the collection 5,000–10,000 U of diluted heparin to help clot dissolution. A larger shielded cannula and application of a manual compression over the collection may also be helpful. A biopsy handle may also be used to obtain a more effective vacuum effect. The collection should be emptied as much as possible. In case of a solid mass, a Tru-Cut needle can be advanced into the lesion and multiple tissue specimens can be collected.

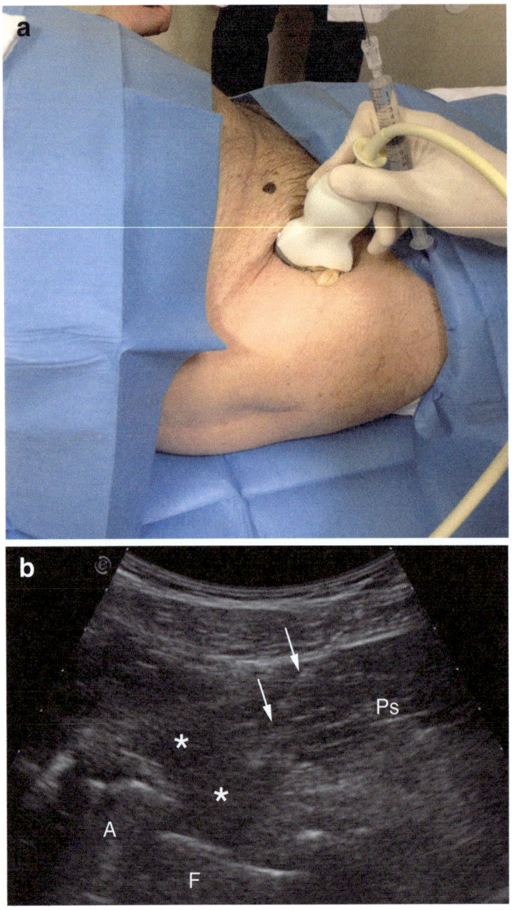

Fig. 5.1 US-guided aspiration of periprosthetic fluid collection. (**a**) Probe and patient position to perform US-guided aspiration of periprosthetic fluid collection using a convex probe. (**b**) US scan of periprosthetic fluid collection aspiration. *Ps* iliopsoas muscle, *A* acetabulum cup, *F* femoral prosthesis, *asterisks* collection, *arrows* needle shaft

STEP 3

In case of periarticular collections, no further actions should be performed. The procedure is shown in **Fig. 5.1**. In case of Morel-Lavallée lesions, compressive bandages should be applied to favor the collapse of the drained cavity. The procedure is shown in **Fig. 5.2**. Local compression is applied anyway and a plaster is placed over the puncture site.

Post-procedure Care

The patient is kept in observation for about 10 min and then discharged from the department.

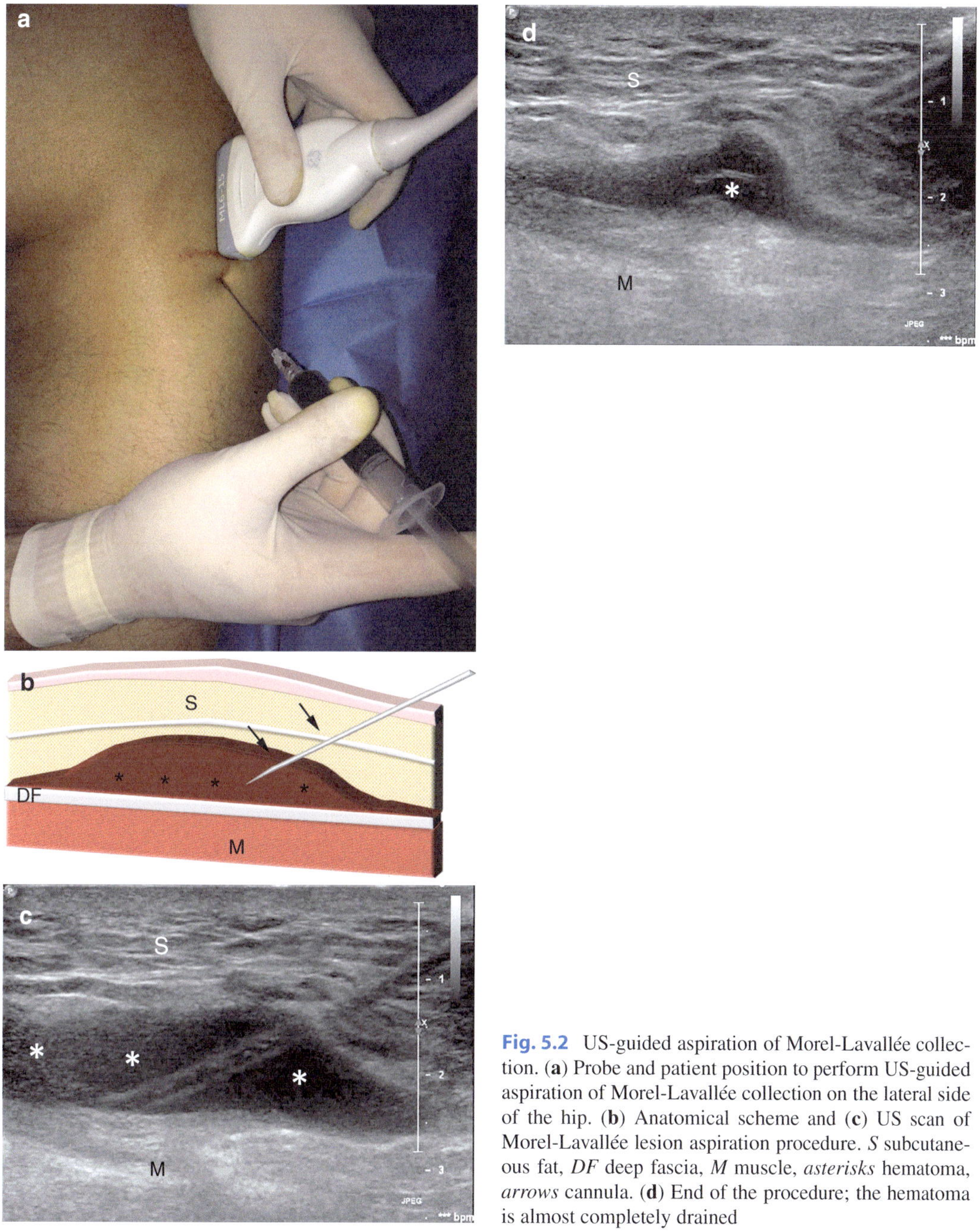

Fig. 5.2 US-guided aspiration of Morel-Lavallée collection. (**a**) Probe and patient position to perform US-guided aspiration of Morel-Lavallée collection on the lateral side of the hip. (**b**) Anatomical scheme and (**c**) US scan of Morel-Lavallée lesion aspiration procedure. *S* subcutaneous fat, *DF* deep fascia, *M* muscle, *asterisks* hematoma, *arrows* cannula. (**d**) End of the procedure; the hematoma is almost completely drained

Bursitis and Cysts Around the Hip

6

Davide Orlandi and Silvia Perugin Bernardi

Essentials

Synovial bursae are anatomical structures that are located in critical regions where tendons run in close relationship with other tendons or bones and act as friction attenuators between such structures during movement. Several bursae are located around the hip: the iliopsoas bursa is located in the anterior compartment between the distal myotendinous junction of the iliopsoas and the anterior aspect of the hip joint; in the lateral compartment, different bursae are located between the glutei and tensor fasciae latae tendons and trochanteric cortical bone; in the posterior compartment, the ischiogluteal bursa lays between the ischial tuberosity and the deep surface of the gluteus maximus.

D. Orlandi (✉)
Department of Internal Medicine, University of Genova, Genova, Italy
e-mail: theabo@libero.it

S. Perugin Bernardi
Postgraduate school in Radiodiagnostics, University of Genoa, School of Medicine, Genoa, Italy
e-mail: silvy-86-@hotmail.it

Iliopsoas Bursa

The iliopsoas bursa is the largest synovial bursa of the human body that lies between the posterior aspect of the iliopsoas muscle and tendon and the anterior capsule of the hip joint, between the medial femoral vessels and the lateral iliopsoas muscle. This bursa allows for smooth gliding between these structures during hip movements. It may present a direct communication with the articular space in up to 15 % of cases, and in normal conditions, it cannot be demonstrated as it contains only a small amount of fluid.

Iliopsoas bursitis often comes along inflammatory or degenerative hip diseases, although it may also represent an isolated primary pathologic condition or a sport-related overuse syndrome. Also, idiopathic bursitis is occasionally described. The iliopsoas bursa may become also extremely large and may occasionally extend in the abdomen through the inguinal canal, mimicking a pelvic lesion.

Peritrochanteric Bursae

A smooth gliding between gluteal and tensor fasciae latae myotendinous structures and trochanteric bone is ensured by the presence of a number of bursae around the greater trochanter. Among them, the most important are the trochanteric

L.M. Sconfienza et al. (eds.), *Ultrasound-guided Musculoskeletal Procedures: The Lower Limb*, DOI 10.1007/978-88-470-5764-7_6

bursa and the bursae of the gluteus medius and minimus.

The large trochanteric bursa is the most constantly present and lays over the lateral aspect of the greater trochanter and the tendon of the gluteus medius.

The bursa of the gluteus medius is located between the anterosuperior part of the lateral facet of the greater trochanter and the gluteus medius tendon.

The gluteus minimus bursa is found anteromedially to the insertion of the gluteus minimus.

Ischiogluteal Bursa

The posterior ischiogluteal bursa is an inconstant, adventitial bursa located in soft tissues between the ischial tuberosity and the deep surface of the gluteus maximus. It is usually not visible and may become distended along with degenerative pathology of hamstrings tendons.

Paralabral Cyst

Similarly to what happens in the shoulder, the acetabulum is surrounded by a triangular-shaped, fibrocartilaginous labrum. Differently from the shoulder, this labrum is uncommonly damaged during trauma, as hip dislocations are extremely unfrequent. However, degenerative joint disease and femoroacetabular impingement may frequently lead to the development of labral fragmentation or tears, particularly over the anterolateral aspect. Here, paralabral cysts may develop, similarly to what happens in the knee with parameniscal cysts. These cysts may remarkably enlarge and mimic a space-occupying mass, which occasionally may extend in the abdomen through the inguinal canal.

Clinical Presentation

When distention and inflammation of a bursal structure is present, symptoms can worsen with pressure of the probe and can vary with certain active and passive movements.

A large distention of the iliopsoas bursitis can lead to symptoms referred in the lower right quadrant of the abdomen, mimicking appendicopathy or pelvic disorders. The same symptoms may be present in conjunction with a large paralabral cyst.

Patients affected by trochanteric bursitis often refer night pain when they sleep on the affected side.

When ischiogluteal bursitis is present, patients often refer pain over the midline of the buttock irradiating caudally along the hamstrings. Prolonged sitting on hard surfaces, repetitive sport movements stressing the ischiogluteal bursa through the hamstring tendon, and severe weight loss (e.g., cachexia) are the main causes which lead to repetitive microtraumas and consequent inflammation of the bursa.

Since the sciatic and the posterior femoral cutaneous nerves run in close contact with this bursa, the inflammation of such structure may also produce symptoms mimicking a radiculopathy.

In all cases, if fever is present, the diagnosis of septic bursitis must be considered.

Ultrasound Diagnosis

Ultrasound can easily detect distention of the bursae around the hip, demonstrating a well-defined anechoic fluid collection between gliding anatomical structures. The pressure applied on the probe determines the squeezing of fluid bursal distentions, helping to differentiate bursitis from other pathological conditions, such as paralabral cysts, which mucinous content is not compressible. Bursal walls can thicken in chronic cases, or internal echogenicity can be present in rheumatic patients due to the presence of a synovial hypertrophy.

Iliopsoas bursitis is seen as an ovoidal, well-defined hypoechoic collection between the medial femoral vessels and the lateral iliopsoas muscle. Paralabral cysts usually have a similar appearance.

Trochanteric bursitis appears as a well-defined, crescentic-shaped hypo-anechoic fluid collection located superficially to the posterior insertion of the gluteus medius and the lateral aspect of the greater trochanter.

Ischiogluteal bursitis is a less frequent condition and can be depicted by US as a superficial, hypo-anechoic fluid collection with lobulated margins (since the adventitial origin of such structure) and thick walls located between the ischial tuberosity tendinous insertion of the hamstrings and the skin when the hips are flexed.

Treatment Options

Conservative treatment includes rest, weight loss, physical therapy, ice, and anti-inflammatory and analgesic medications. US-guided aspiration and subsequent steroid injection is necessary in the case of symptomatic, large bursal or cystic distension. Infections in this area are uncommon but may be present in case of septic arthritis, particularly after hip prosthesis. In these cases, US-guided aspiration and microbiological analysis of the bursal fluid is required before starting antibiotic therapy.

Interventional Procedure

Indications

Diagnostic aspiration or therapeutic pain relief. Intra-bursal or intra-cystic injection of steroids. Contraindicated if suspected or known bursal infection or in the presence of overlying cellulitis or infection, hypersensitivity to corticosteroids.

Objective

To aspirate fluid and to deliver anti-inflammatory drugs within the bursa/cyst.

Equipment

- 1 syringe (20 ml)
- 16–18 G needle
- Long-acting steroid (1 ml, 40 mg/ml)
- Plaster

How We Do It

STEP 1

The patient is positioned in a different way according to the bursa to treat, and a US scan is made to identify the enlarged bursa and to assess its anatomical extension.

Iliopsoas bursitis or paralabral cyst: the patient lies in supine position with the lower limb slightly extra-rotated. The bursa or the cyst is well demonstrated by means of a parasagittal scan, and the needle can be inserted with an in-plane caudo-cranial approach to reach the bursal/cyst space. The procedure is shown in Fig. 6.1.

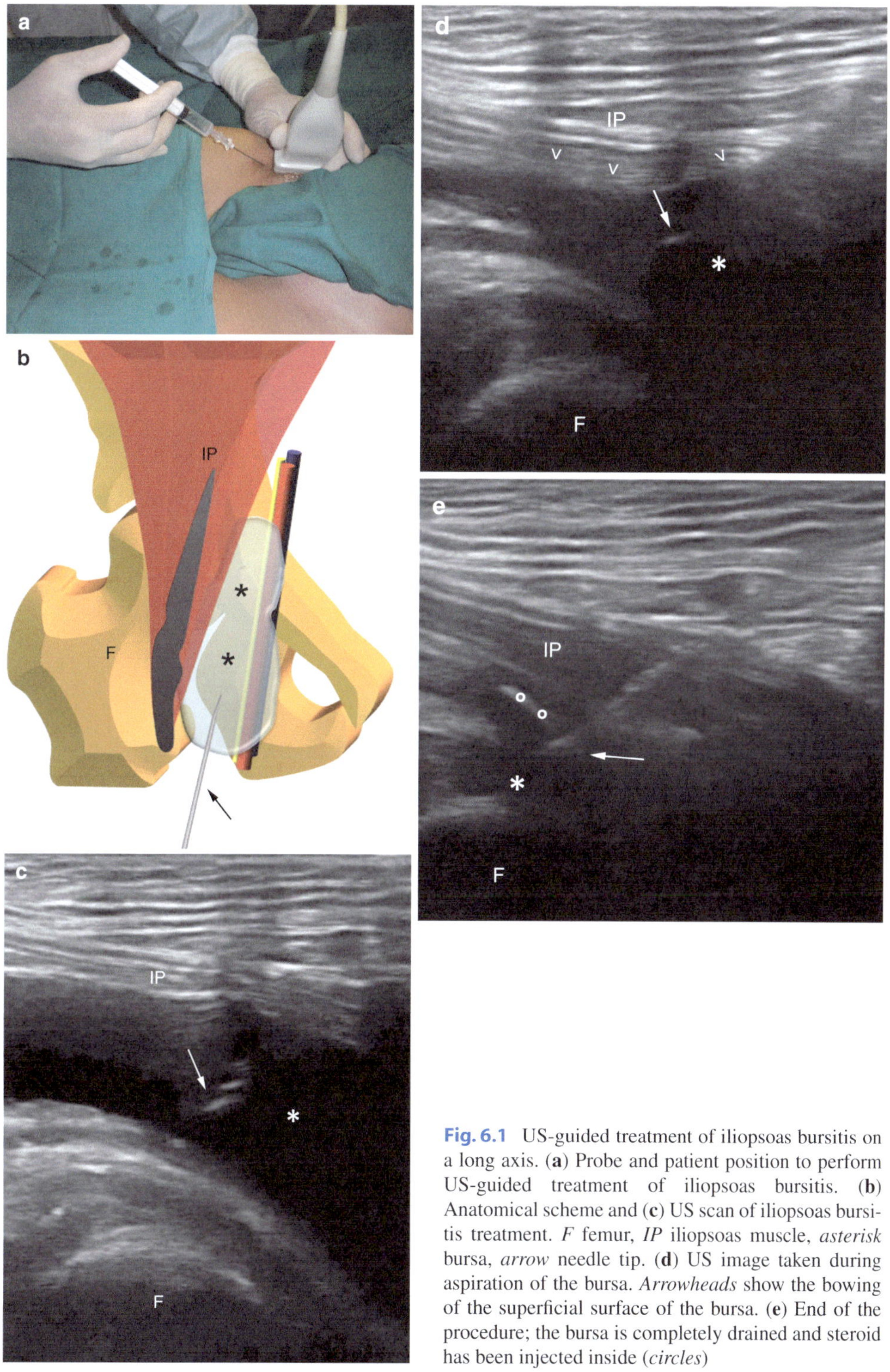

Fig. 6.1 US-guided treatment of iliopsoas bursitis on a long axis. (**a**) Probe and patient position to perform US-guided treatment of iliopsoas bursitis. (**b**) Anatomical scheme and (**c**) US scan of iliopsoas bursitis treatment. *F* femur, *IP* iliopsoas muscle, *asterisk* bursa, *arrow* needle tip. (**d**) US image taken during aspiration of the bursa. *Arrowheads* show the bowing of the superficial surface of the bursa. (**e**) End of the procedure; the bursa is completely drained and steroid has been injected inside (*circles*)

Peritrochanteric bursitis: the patient lies on the contralateral side. The bursa is demonstrated with an axial scan over the greater trochanter avoiding applying excessive pressure. The needle can be inserted with a posterior-to-anterior, medial-to-lateral, in-plane approach. In the case of distention of the gluteus medius or minimus bursae, an anterior-to-posterior insertion of the needle is necessary. The procedure is shown in Fig. 6.2.

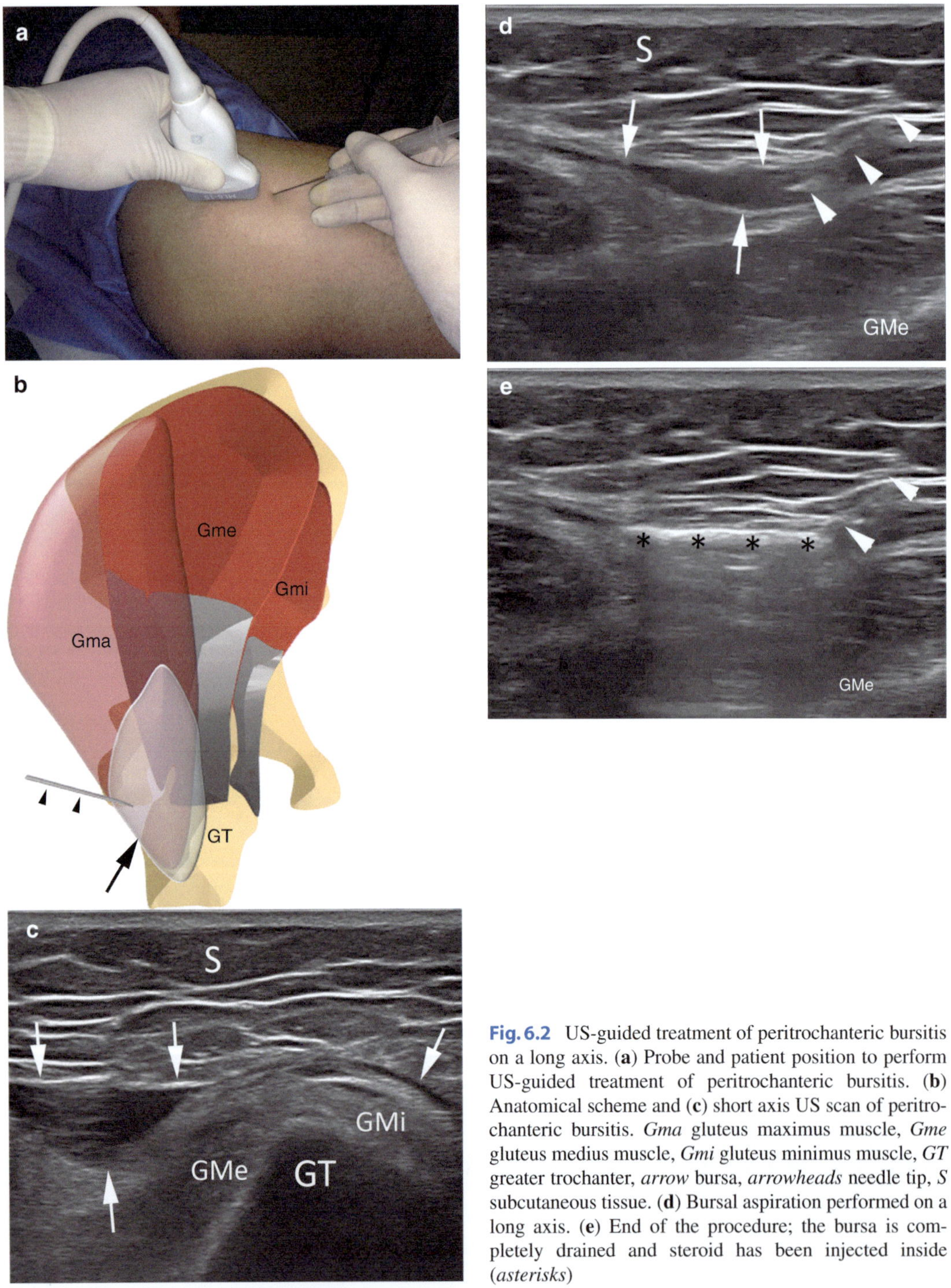

Fig. 6.2 US-guided treatment of peritrochanteric bursitis on a long axis. (**a**) Probe and patient position to perform US-guided treatment of peritrochanteric bursitis. (**b**) Anatomical scheme and (**c**) short axis US scan of peritrochanteric bursitis. *Gma* gluteus maximus muscle, *Gme* gluteus medius muscle, *Gmi* gluteus minimus muscle, *GT* greater trochanter, *arrow* bursa, *arrowheads* needle tip, *S* subcutaneous tissue. (**d**) Bursal aspiration performed on a long axis. (**e**) End of the procedure; the bursa is completely drained and steroid has been injected inside (*asterisks*)

Ischiogluteal bursitis: the patient is positioned prone and the bursal structure is demonstrated by means of a parasagittal US scan. The needle can be inserted with an in-plane, caudal-to-cranial approach.

STEP 2

A needle connected to a syringe is inserted with an in-plane approach until the needle tip enters the bursa or cyst. The content may be very dense and drainage could be extremely challenging. In these cases, the operator may inject in the bursa or in the cyst a small amount of lidocaine (5 ml) to dilute the content and aspirate it more easily. A larger shielded cannula and application of a manual compression over the bursa may also be helpful. A biopsy handle may also be used to obtain a more effective vacuum effect.

STEP 3

When the bursa or cyst is completely drained, a small amount of steroid (1 ml) is then injected. This has the purpose of both reducing inflammation and helping the walls to remain collapsed. The needle is then removed, local compression is applied, and a plaster is placed over the puncture site.

Post-procedure Care

The patient is kept in observation for about 10 min. Pain after treatment may occasionally occur and it could be managed using oral NSAIDs.

Part II

The Knee

7 The Knee: Focused Ultrasound Anatomy and Examination Technique

Riccardo Sartoris and Angelo Corazza

The knee can be divided into four compartments, anterior, medial, lateral, and posterior.

Anterior Compartment

Anatomy

The quadriceps tendon is formed by four independent slips that come from the four muscles composing the quadriceps muscle, namely, the rectus femoris, vastus lateralis, vastus intermedius, and vastus medialis. The four slips are interspersed with thin fat and connective layers and conjoined in a single tendon that inserts over the proximal pole of the patella. Under the quadriceps tendon, the suprapatellar joint recess can be seen. This space is particularly useful to perform ultrasound-guided intra-articular injections.

The patellar tendon (or ligament) arises from the inferior pole of the patella, courses longitudinally, and inserts distally over the anterior tibial apophysis.

Scanning Technique

The patient lays on the bed with the lower limb extended and the knee 30° to 45° flexed. A pillow or a cylindrical support may be placed under the popliteal fossa to support the knee during the examination. The probe should be placed on a longitudinal plane over the proximal pole of the patella that can be easily palpated and sled proximal to encounter the patellar tendon. Then, the probe should be sled distally and the patellar tendon evaluated with longitudinal scans up to the anterior tibial apophysis. Attention should be paid to tendon insertions, as the deepest portion may be affected by anisotropy (Figs. 7.1 and 7.2).

R. Sartoris (✉) • A. Corazza
Postgraduate school in Radiodiagnostics, University of Genoa, School of Medicine, Genoa, Italy
e-mail: riccardo.sartoris@hotmail.it; angelcoraz@libero.it

L.M. Sconfienza et al. (eds.), *Ultrasound-guided Musculoskeletal Procedures: The Lower Limb*, DOI 10.1007/978-88-470-5764-7_7

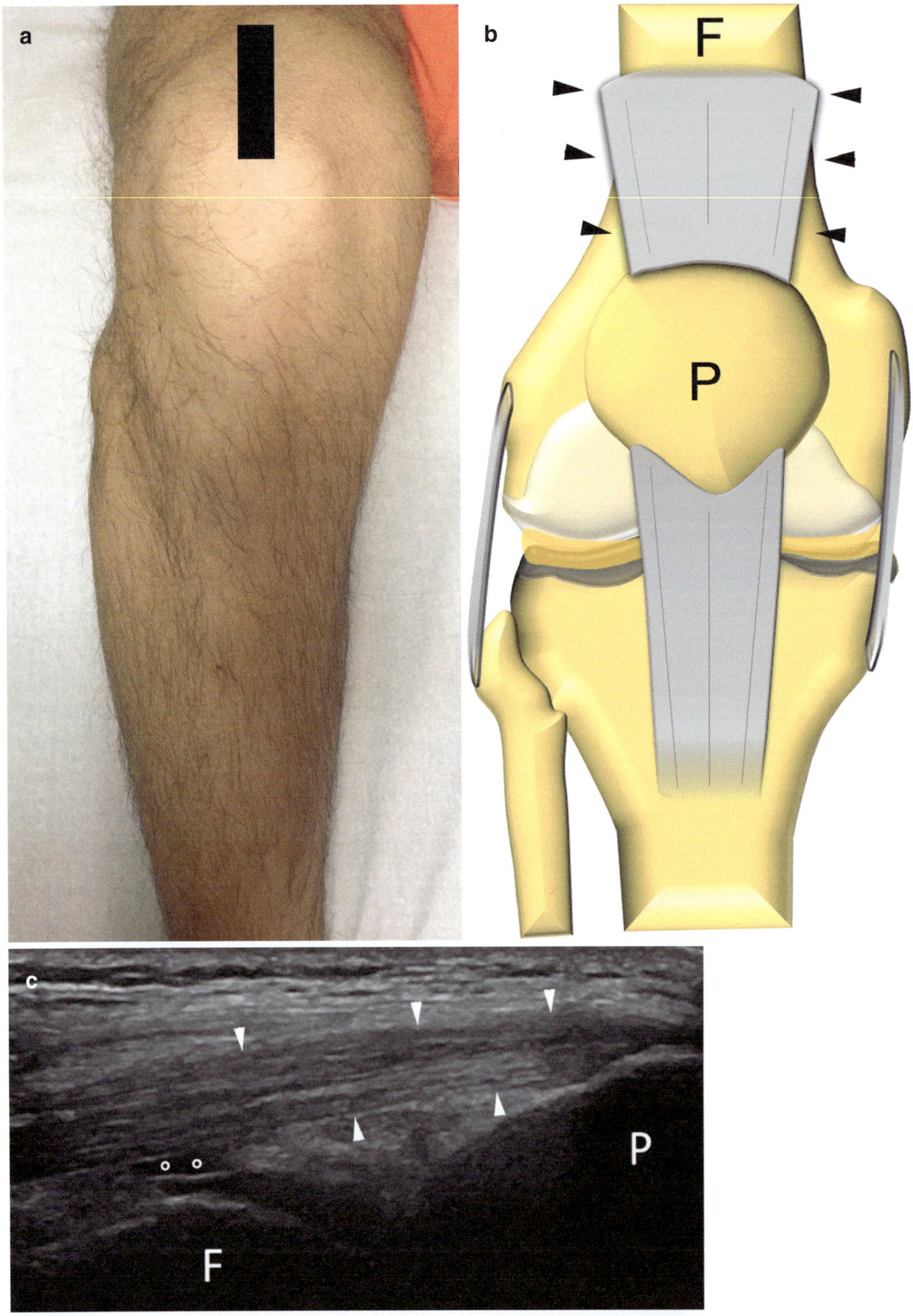

Fig. 7.1 Evaluation of the anterior knee to assess the quadriceps tendon and the suprapatellar joint recess. (**a**) The probe and patient are positioned to evaluate the quadriceps tendon and the suprapatellar joint recess on a long-axis scan. (**b**) Anatomical scheme of the quadriceps tendon and the suprapatellar joint recess as seen frontally. *F* femoris, *P* patella, *arrowheads* quadriceps tendon, *circles* suprapatellar joint recess. (**c**) US long-axis scan of the quadriceps tendon and the suprapatellar joint recess

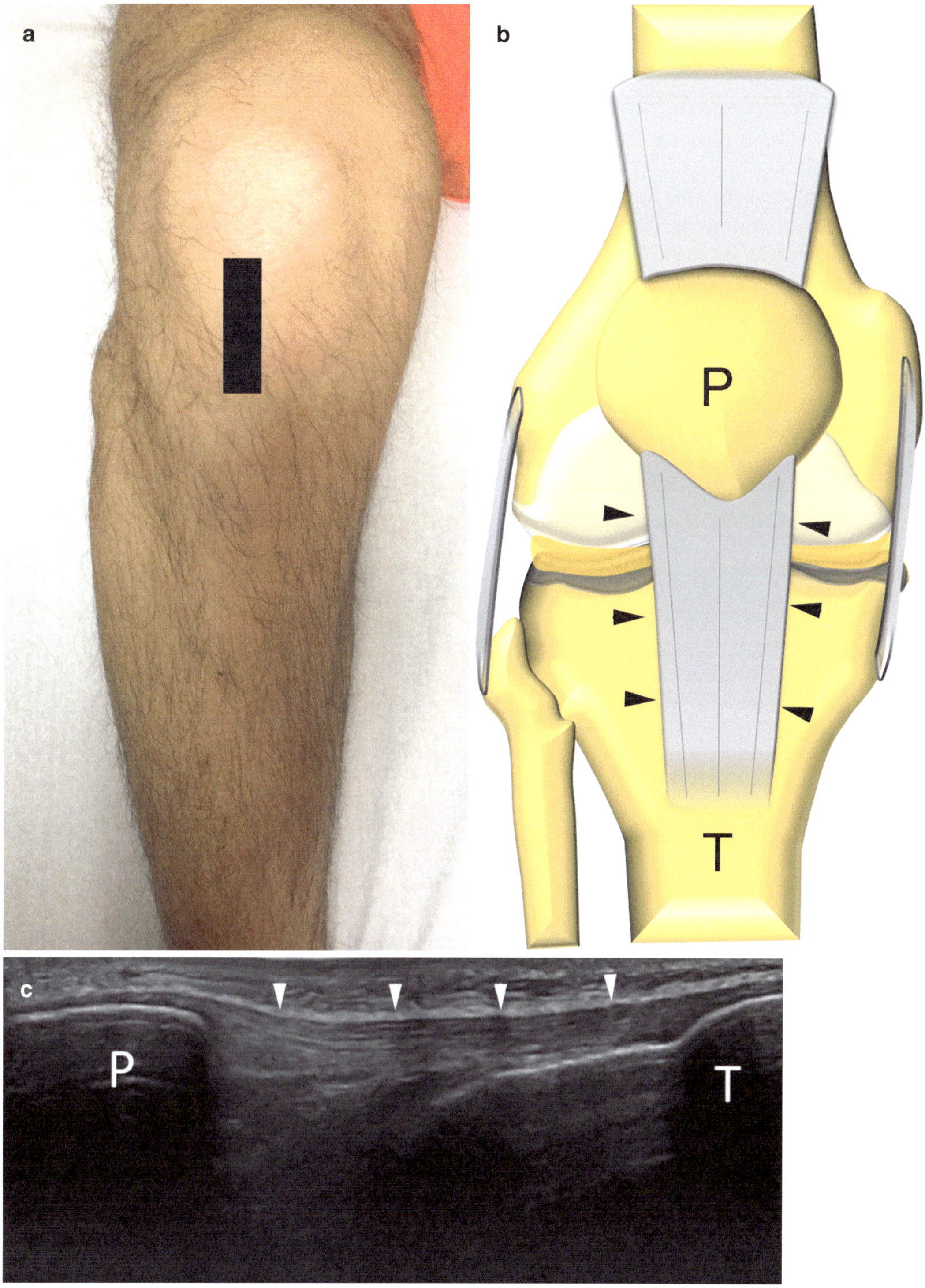

Fig. 7.2 Evaluation of the anterior knee to assess the patellar tendon. (**a**) The probe and patient are positioned to evaluate the patellar tendon on a long-axis scan. (**b**) Anatomical scheme of the patellar tendon as seen frontally. *T* tibia, *P* patella, *arrowheads* patellar tendon. (**c**) US long-axis scan of the patellar tendon

Medial Compartment

Anatomy

The medial collateral ligament is a band-like ligament that courses oblique from the medial aspect of the femoral condyle to the medial aspect of the tibia. Slightly anterior to the distal attachment of the medial collateral ligament, the insertion of the three tendons of the goose's foot can be seen, namely, sartorius, gracilis, and semitendinosus. The tendons are surrounded by the goose's foot bursa, which cannot be seen when not distended.

Scanning Technique

The knee is positioned similarly to what was reported for the examination of the anterior compartment. The probe is placed on a coronal oblique plane to detect the double-layered appearance of the medial collateral ligament. Then, the probe should be sled more distally and anteriorly to perform a longitudinal scan of the goose's foot tendons. Of note, if the goose's foot bursa is not distended, the tendons can be scarcely differentiated one from the other (Fig. 7.3).

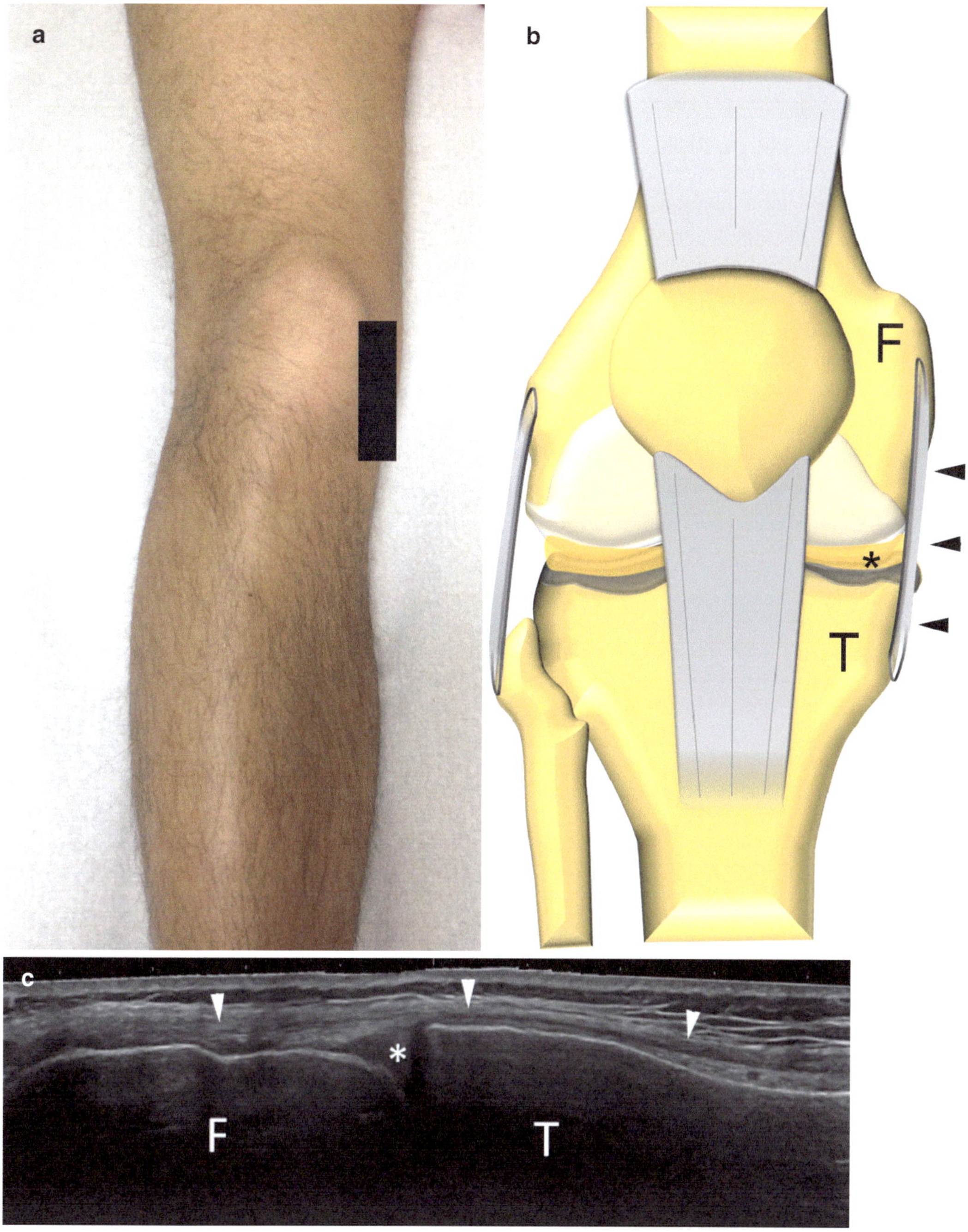

Fig. 7.3 Evaluation of the medial knee. (**a**) The probe and patient are positioned to evaluate the medial knee on a long-axis scan. (**b**) Anatomical scheme of the medial knee. *T* tibia, *F* femur, *arrowheads* medial collateral ligament, *asterisk* medial meniscus. (**c**) US long-axis scan of the medial knee

Lateral Compartment

Anatomy

The lateral collateral ligament is a cord-like, fibrillar structure that runs over the lateral knee. It attaches on the lateral femoral condyle proximally and over the fibular head distally. More anteriorly, the iliotibial band can be seen, attaching distally over the Gerdy's tubercle.

The common peroneal nerve is a branch of the sciatic nerve that arises proximally to the popliteal fossa. The common peroneal nerve courses distally around the fibular head, where it can be impinged, and further subdivides into two branches, the superficial peroneal and the deep peroneal nerve.

Scanning Technique

The lateral collateral ligament is better evaluated with the knee flexed 45° to 60°. The probe should be oriented on a coronal oblique plane with one edge over the fibular head. Moving the probe more anteriorly allows for evaluating the iliotibial band, approximately with the same orientation. The common peroneal nerve is usually evaluated with axial scans over the fibular head, sliding the probe proximal to distal. The nerve is seen turning around the fibular head, from posterior to anterior (Figs. 7.4 and 7.5).

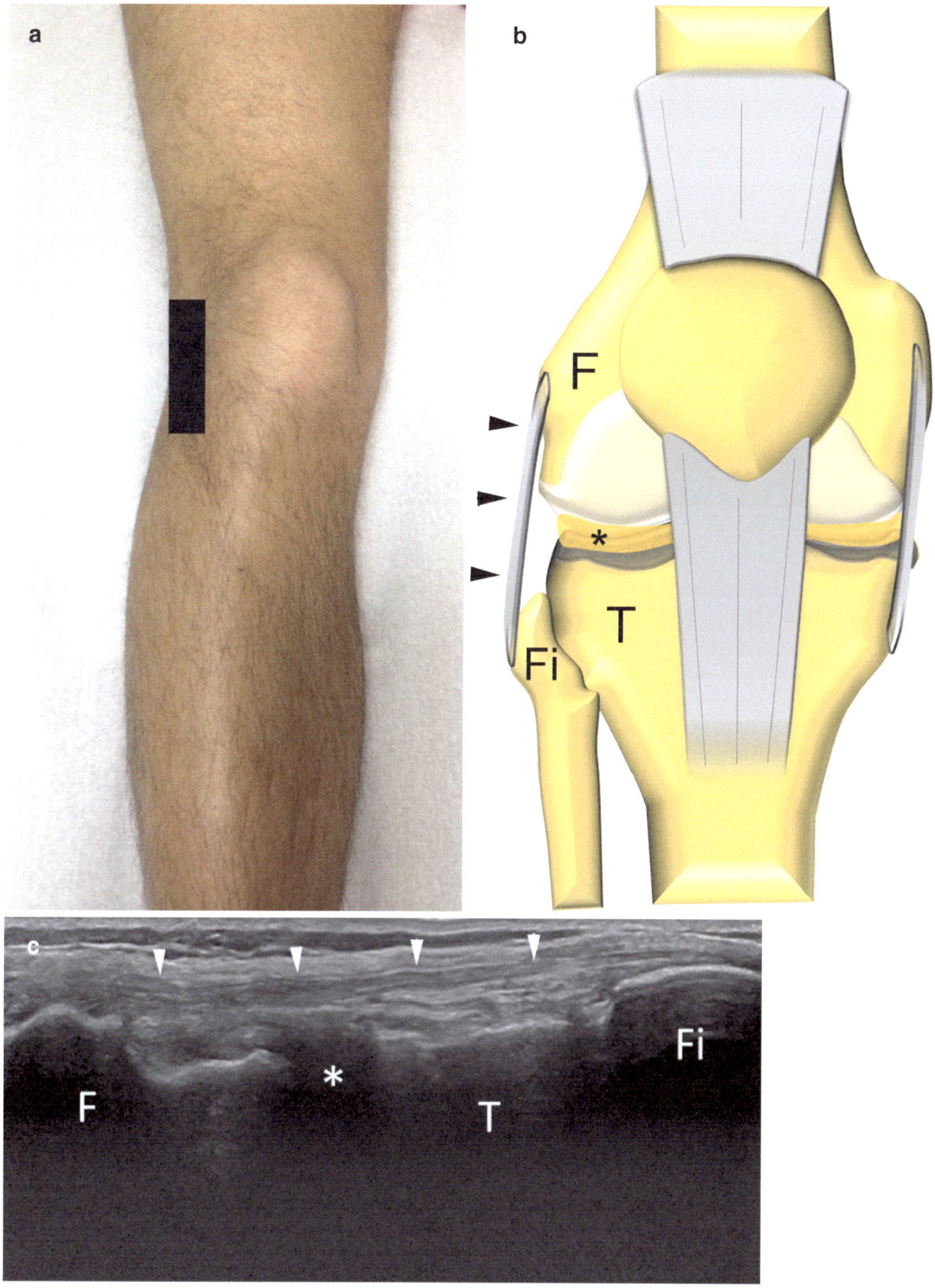

Fig. 7.4 Evaluation of the lateral knee. (**a**) The probe and patient are positioned to evaluate the lateral on a long-axis scan. (**b**) Anatomical scheme of the lateral knee. *Ti* tibia, *F* femur, *Fi* fibula, *arrowheads* lateral collateral ligament, *asterisk* lateral meniscus. (**c**) US long-axis scan of the lateral knee

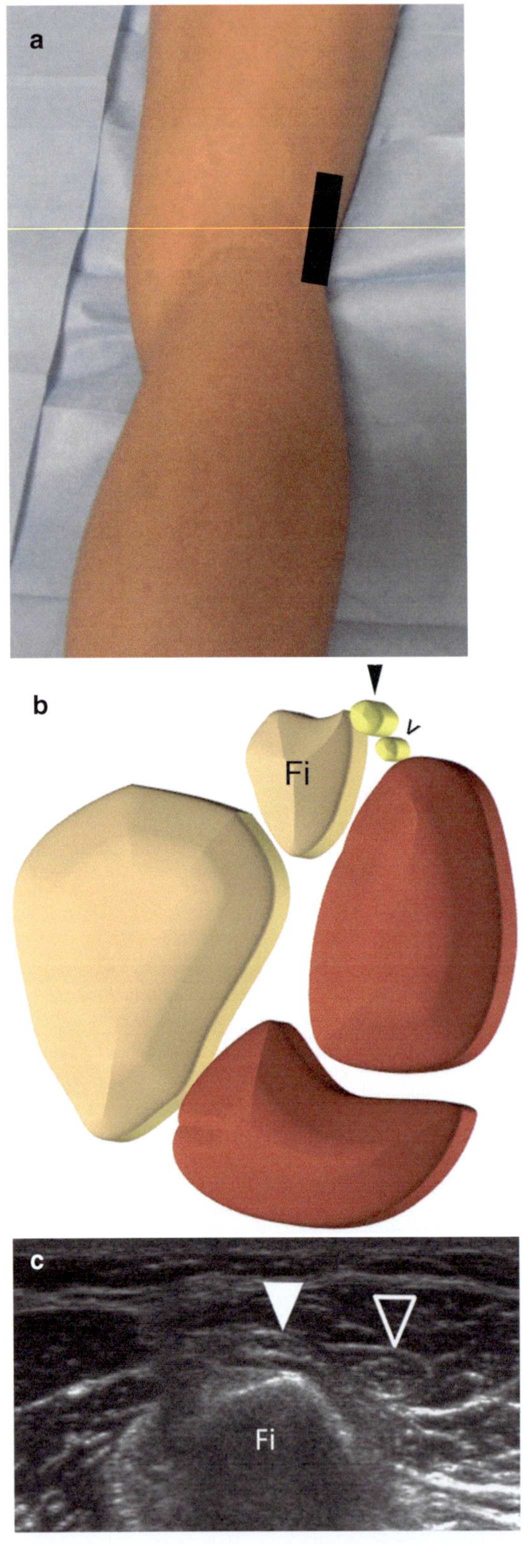

Fig. 7.5 Evaluation of the peroneal nerve. (**a**) The probe and patient are positioned to evaluate the peroneal nerve on a short-axis scan. (**b**) Anatomical scheme of the peroneal nerve as seen along its short axis. *Fi* fibula, *open arrowhead* deep branch of the peroneal nerve, *solid arrowhead* superficial branch of the peroneal nerve. (**c**) US short-axis scan of the branches of the peroneal nerve around the fibula

Posterior Compartment

Anatomy

The posterior compartment of the knee mainly contains muscular structures. The semimembranosus is a long muscle arising from the ischial tuberosity, inserting distally over the posterior tibial condyle. Between the semimembranosus and the medial gastrocnemius muscle, the semimembranosus bursa can be seen with a typical C shape. The bursa has a communication with the joint space in more than half of cases.

Scanning Technique

The patient should be positioned prone over the bed with the knee fully extended. The area between the medial gastrocnemius muscle and semimembranosus tendon can be seen by placing the probe on the medial side of the popliteal fossa. When not distended, the bursa is not directly visible. Conversely, a pathologic bursa is usually filled with anechoic synovial fluid. The distended bursa may also be seen with iso-/hyperechoic appearance, when synovial hypertrophy is present (Fig. 7.6).

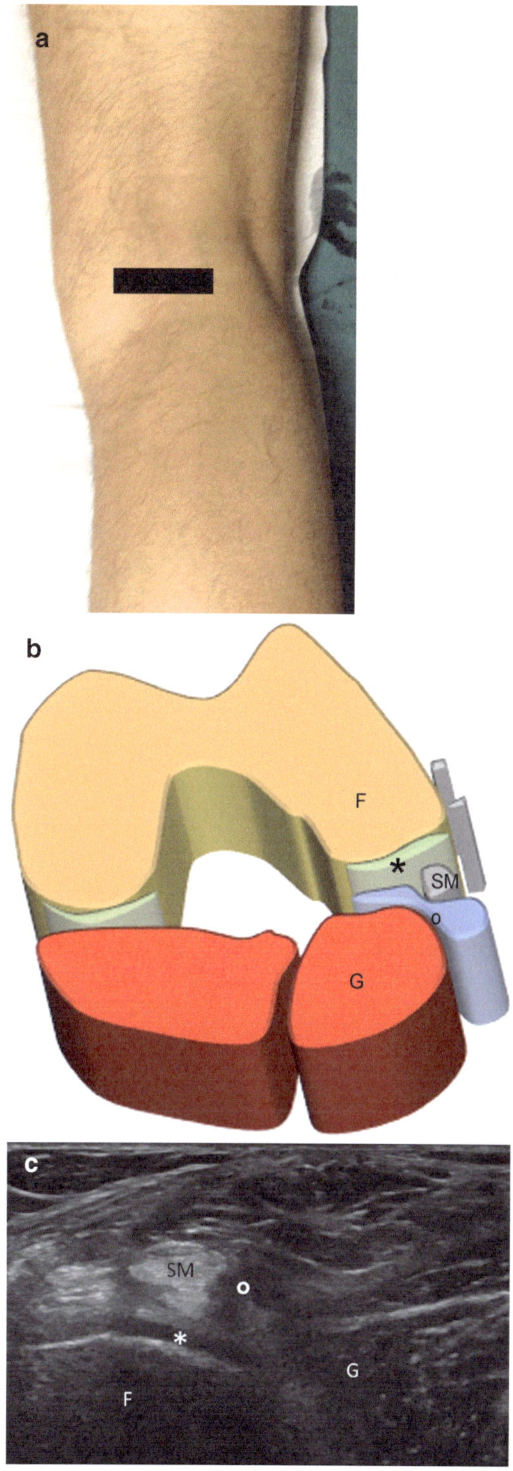

Fig. 7.6 Evaluation of the posterior medial knee. (**a**) The probe and patient are positioned to evaluate the posterior medial knee on a short-axis scan. (**b**) Anatomical scheme of the posterior medial knee as seen along its short axis. *F* femur, *asterisk* femoral cartilage, *SM* semimembranosus, *G* gastrocnemius, *circle* gastrocnemius-semimembranosus bursa. (**c**) US short-axis scan of the posterior medial knee

Knee Intra-articular Injections

8

Giovanni Serafini and Francesca Lacelli

Essentials

Intra-articular injections of the knee can be performed to treat a number of pathologic conditions. The drugs administered in these cases may be anti-inflammatory agents, such as steroids, that may be indicated for patients with advanced hip osteoarthritis (OA) refractory to other treatments or viscosupplements, such as hyaluronic acid, that can be used to treat patients with mild to moderate OA. Anesthetics may be injected in conjunction to steroids but are not routinely used for diagnostic purposes.

Knee OA

Knee OA is a very common condition, affecting up to 13 % of women and 10 % of men over 60 years. Primary knee OA is a degenerative joint disease frequently associated with aging and increased loads on this weight-bearing joint, two conditions that frequently coexist. Secondary knee OA can be found in patients with untreated lower limb malalignment or patients with previous fractures, in which altered biomechanics usually lead to joint damage.

G. Serafini (✉) • F. Lacelli
Unit of Radiology, Ospedale Santa Corona,
ASL 2 Savonese, Pietra Ligure, Italy
e-mail: giovanni.serafini52@gmail.com;
francy78@libero.it

Clinical Presentation

The main symptom is usually joint pain that occurs during the whole day. Joint stiffness may be variably associated with pain, swelling, or tenderness in the knee joint and inability to perform routine activities. Occasionally, a sound or feeling of bone rubbing against bone is reported.

Ultrasound Diagnosis

The diagnosis of knee OA requires plain film examination. However, US can demonstrate the presence of joint effusion, osteophytes over the external edges of the tibia and the femur, and extruded, inhomogeneous menisci. Magnetic resonance imaging may be required to detect the presence of associated abnormalities.

Treatment Options

Conservative treatment includes weight loss, physical therapy, oral anti-inflammatory and analgesic medications, and intra-articular injections (hyaluronic acid, steroids). At later stage, monocompartmental prosthesis or total knee replacement can be implanted.

L.M. Sconfienza et al. (eds.), *Ultrasound-guided Musculoskeletal Procedures: The Lower Limb*, DOI 10.1007/978-88-470-5764-7_8

Interventional Procedure

Indications

Painful primary or secondary OA, conservative treatment in patients ineligible for total hip arthroplasty: hyaluronic acid or steroid injection.

Inflammatory arthritis: steroid injection.

Intra-articular injections are generally contraindicated in patients with suspected or known joint infection, overlying cellulitis, or hypersensitivity to the pertinent drug.

This procedure can also be used to inject contrast agents within the joint for arthrography purposes.

Objective

To deliver anti-inflammatory or viscosupplementant drugs within the joint space.

Equipment

- 1 syringe (2–5 ml)
- 20 G spinal needle
- Long-acting steroid (1 ml, 40 mg/ml) or hyaluronic acid (2–6 ml)
- Plaster

How We Do It

Intra-articular knee injections are reported to be relatively easy when performed using superficial bony landmarks as references. Also, the absence of any potentially dangerous structure makes this procedure even safer and easier. However, it has been reported that up to 40 % of blinded injections do not reach the target. Thus, ultrasound guidance definitely improves injection accuracy. At the level of the hip is generally more complex when compared to other joints (e.g., shoulder, knee) for its deep location and the relative contiguity of the femoral neurovascular bundle.

Lateral (in-plane) approach is normally used for this procedure, thus allowing for a direct and continuous visualization of the needle along the whole path in soft tissues. The procedure is shown in Fig. 8.1.

STEP 1

The patient lies in supine position with the knee 30° to 45° flexed. The probe is positioned on an axial scan over the distal insertion of the quadriceps tendon and then sled slightly laterally to visualize the tendon medially and the lateral joint recess laterally. A variable amount of fluid and synovial hypertrophy can be seen in the recess. This usually helps to have the recess more distended and to visualize the target more reliably.

STEP 2

With the articular recess centered in the middle of the screen, a 20 G needle is inserted from the lateral side of the probe. Whatever the knee size, the needle should be usually inserted more or less parallel to the probe. With this approach, the whole path of the needle can be visualized in real time and slight corrections of the direction can be made. In case of abundant joint effusion, it should be aspirated before injecting any drug, as this may improve the efficacy of the procedure. Then, the drug can be injected.

STEP 3

At the end of the injection, the needle can be removed and a plaster should be applied.

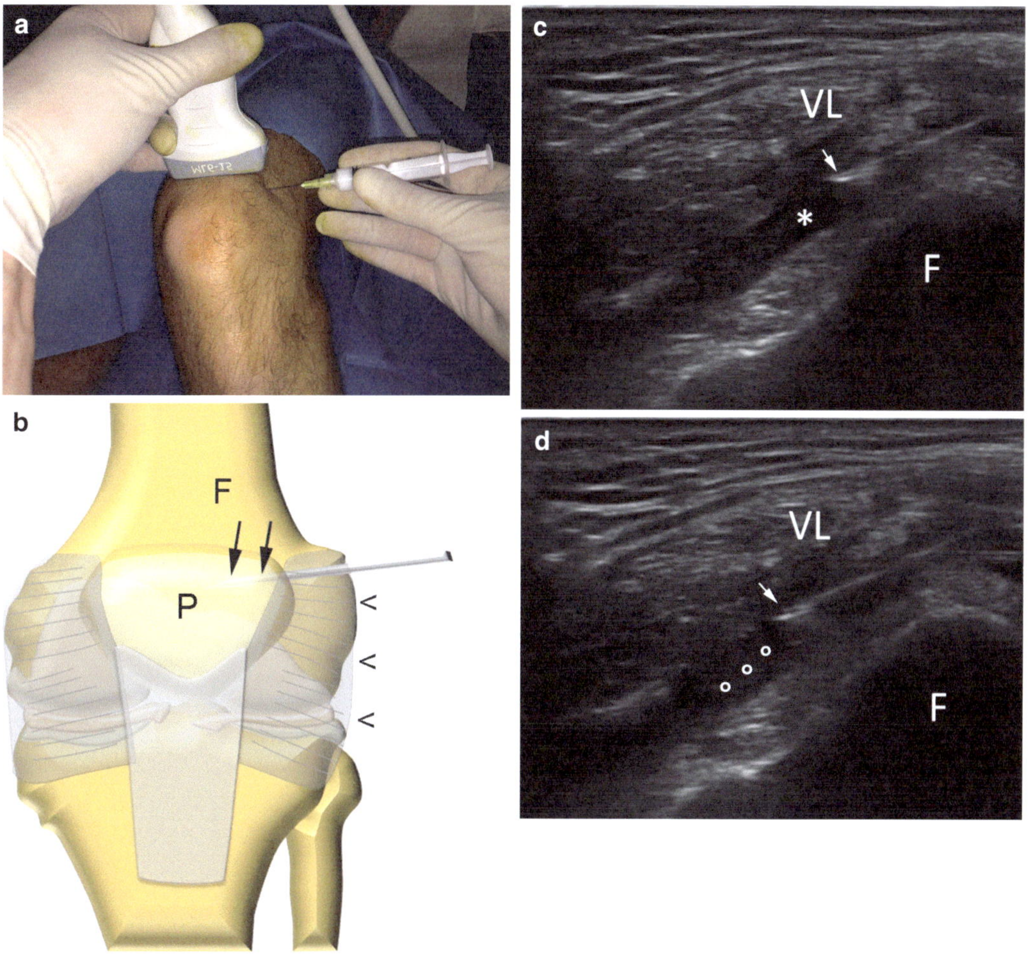

Fig. 8.1 US-guided intra-articular knee injection on a short axis. (**a**) Probe and patient position to perform short-axis US-guided intra-articular knee injection. (**b**) Anatomical scheme and (**c**) US scan of short-axis intra-articular knee injection. *P* patella, *F* femur, *arrowheads* lateral joint capsule, *asterisk* suprapatellar joint recess, *arrows* needle, *VL* vastus lateralis. (**d**) US scan showing steroid (*circles*) intra-articular injection

Post-procedural Care

The patient is usually kept under observation for about 10 min after the procedure. Pain may occur after treatment and can be managed with a short course of oral NSAIDs.

Bursitis and Cysts Around the Knee

9

Angelo Corazza and Riccardo Sartoris

Essentials

Synovial bursae are anatomical structures that are located in critical regions where tendons run in close relationship with other tendons or bones and act as friction attenuators between such structures during movement. In the knee, several bursae can be found, but three of them are those mostly commonly involved by pathologic conditions: the bursa between the medial gastrocnemius muscle and the semimembranosus tendon, the goose's foot bursa, and the prepatellar bursa.

Cysts may arise in different locations around the knee, parameniscal cysts being the most common.

Gastrocnemius-Semimembranosus Bursa

The gastrocnemius-semimembranosus bursa is a C-shaped bursa that is designed to reduce the friction between the medial gastrocnemius muscle and the semimembranosus tendon prior to its insertion over the tibia. Primary pathologic involvement of this bursa is relatively uncommon. However, a bursitis is frequently associated to degenerative knee disease and, particularly, to tears of the posterior horn of the medial meniscus, which may allow for direct joint communication. This bursa may become extremely enlarged and assume a cystic appearance, not infrequently containing cartilage debris (e.g., osteochondral bodies) and synovial hypertrophy. In patients with inflammatory joint disease, the cystic appearance of the bursa is also known as "Baker's cyst."

Parameniscal Cysts

Meniscal tears are extremely frequent, both in young athletes in whom trauma is usually the main cause and in elderly subjects in whom menisci are usually degenerated. Parameniscal cysts (or ganglia) may arise from these tears, especially those located over the anterior horn of the lateral meniscus. They may be very small and only incidentally detected during routine magnetic resonance examination but may also reach large dimensions. When lateral, these cysts may also develop within the fascicles of the intra-articular branch of the superficial peroneal nerve.

A. Corazza (✉) • R. Sartoris
Postgraduate School in Radiodiagnostics, University of Genova, School of Medicine, Genoa, Italy
e-mail: angelcoraz@libero.it;
riccardo.sartoris@hotmail.it

L.M. Sconfienza et al. (eds.), *Ultrasound-guided Musculoskeletal Procedures: The Lower Limb*, DOI 10.1007/978-88-470-5764-7_9

Goose's Foot Bursa

The goose's foot bursa has the function to reduce friction between the three tendons of this area, namely, the semitendinosus, the gracilis, and the sartorius. Inflammation of this bursa is relatively common in athletes, in whom overuse may cause pain and swelling over the medial aspect of the knee. As medial knee pain is frequently referred to medial meniscus tears, the presence of a goose's foot bursitis may be overlooked.

Prepatellar Bursitis

This pathologic condition is also known as the "housemaid's knee," as it is mainly caused by a continuous and direct friction of the anterior knee over a hard surface (e.g., the floor). Also, it is not infrequent to see elderly patients with a prepatellar bursitis after direct trauma.

Clinical Presentation

When distention and inflammation of a bursal structure is present, symptoms can worsen with pressure of the probe and can vary with certain active and passive movements.

A large cystic distention of the gastrocnemius-semimembranosus bursa may present with a large, hard, elastic lump over the posterior medial aspect of the knee. Of note, gastrocnemius-semimembranosus bursitis may change over time in size, and it may happen that a patient reports the presence of a large lump in the past that is not visible at the moment of the examination.

Being parameniscal cyst associated to meniscal tears, the treatment should be aimed to take care of these latter. However, when parameniscal cysts reach large dimensions, they may cause pain due to space occupation and compression on the surrounding structures. When parameniscal cysts involve the intra-articular branch of the superficial peroneal nerve, neuropathic symptoms are frequent.

Goose's foot bursitis is usually difficult to detect clinically as the pain may mimic the presence of a meniscal tear or of a patellar cartilage degeneration. However, direct pressure over the insertion of the goose's foot tendons may help to orient the diagnosis.

Prepatellar bursitis usually present with pain over the superficial aspect of the patella. When the bursitis is large, a lump may also be present.

Ultrasound Diagnosis

Ultrasound can easily detect distention of the bursae and the presence of cysts around the knee. Bursitis and cysts usually present as well-defined anechoic fluid collection. As reported above, bursitis and cysts may occasionally contain solid tissue that represents synovial proliferation. The pressure applied on the probe determines the squeezing of fluid bursal distentions, helping to differentiate bursitis from other pathologic conditions, such as parameniscal cysts.

Gastrocnemius-semimembranosus bursitis usually appears as a C-shaped, well-defined hypoechoic collection between the medial gastrocnemius muscle and the semimembranosus tendon.

Parameniscal cysts usually present as multilocular, hypoechoic lumps around the femorotibial rim. Although arising from the menisci, the connecting pedicle may not be visible.

Goose's foot bursitis is usually difficult to see when small. When larger, it presents as a thin hypoechoic layer over the three anteromedial tendons.

Prepatellar bursitis is usually a hypoechoic collection over the anterior aspect of the patella. Usually, the walls are very thin and not visible. As traumatic bursitis may contain a certain amount of blood, the detection of hyperechoic clots inside the bursa is not infrequent.

Treatment Options

Conservative treatment includes rest, weight loss, physical therapy, ice, and anti-inflammatory and analgesic medications. US-guided aspiration and subsequent steroid injection are necessary in the case of symptomatic, large bursal, or cystic distension. Infections around the knee are uncommon, with the exception of prepatellar bursitis that may occasionally complicate with superinfection. In these cases, US-guided aspiration and microbiological analysis of the bursal fluid is required before starting antibiotic therapy.

Interventional Procedure

Indications

Diagnostic aspiration or therapeutic pain relief. Intra-bursal or intra-cystic injection of steroids. Contraindicated if suspected or known bursal infection or in the presence of overlying cellulitis or infection and hypersensitivity to corticosteroids.

Objective

To aspirate fluid and to deliver anti-inflammatory drugs within the bursa/cyst

Equipment

- 1 syringe (5–20 ml)
- 16–18 G needle
- Long-acting steroid (1 ml, 40 mg/ml)
- Plaster

STEP 1

The patient is positioned in a different way according to the bursa/cyst to treat, and a US scan is made to identify the structure and to assess its anatomical extension.

Gastrocnemius-semimembranosus bursitis: the patient lies in prone position with the lower limb extended. The bursa is well demonstrated using an axial or a sagittal scan over the medial aspect of the posterior knee. The needle can be inserted with lateral-medial (when axial scan is performed) or caudo-cranial or cranio-caudal approach (when sagittal scan is performed). Note that when using a lateral-medial approach, extreme caution should be taken to avoid the popliteal neurovascular bundle. The procedure is shown in **Fig. 9.1**.

How We Do It

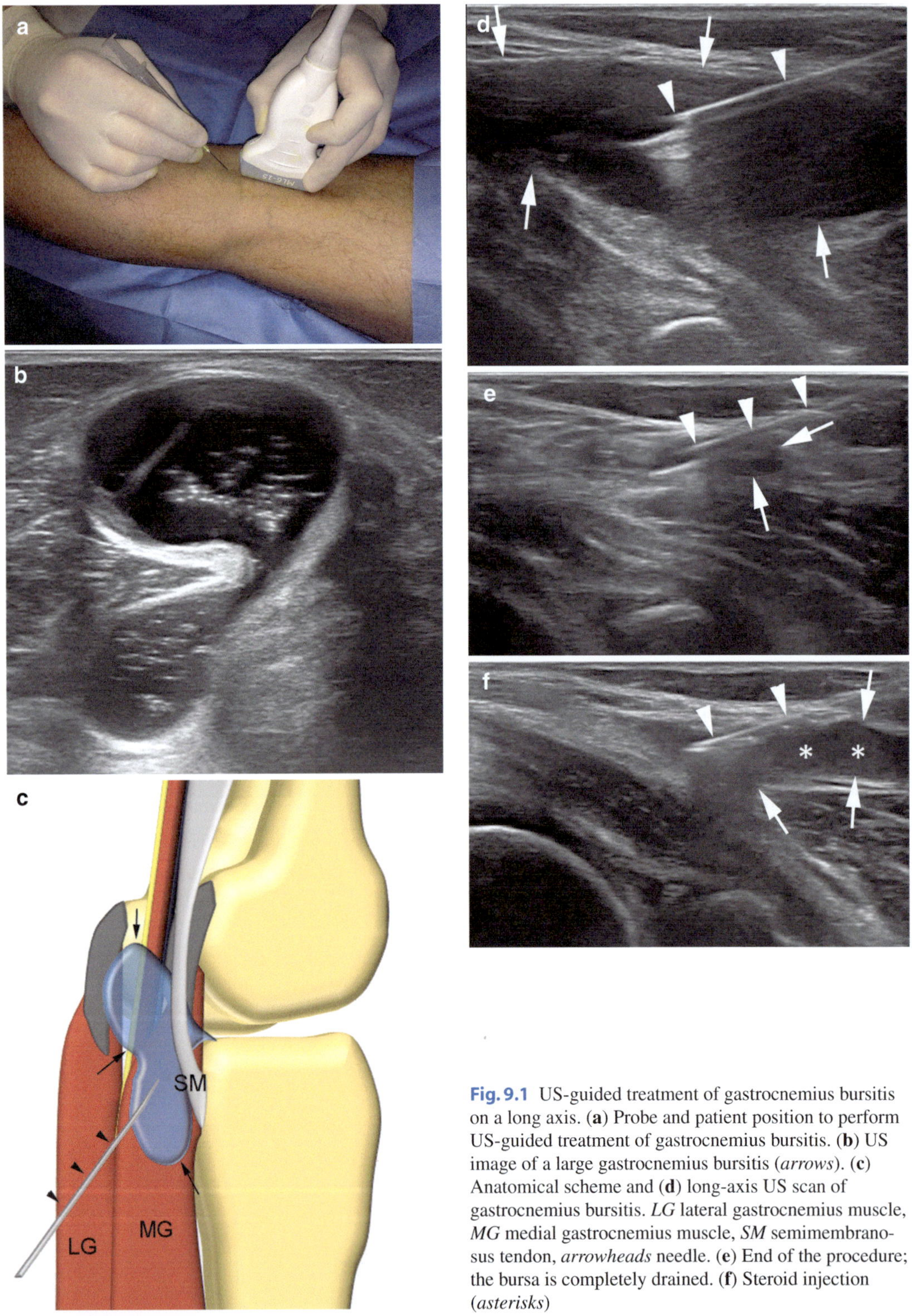

Fig. 9.1 US-guided treatment of gastrocnemius bursitis on a long axis. (**a**) Probe and patient position to perform US-guided treatment of gastrocnemius bursitis. (**b**) US image of a large gastrocnemius bursitis (*arrows*). (**c**) Anatomical scheme and (**d**) long-axis US scan of gastrocnemius bursitis. *LG* lateral gastrocnemius muscle, *MG* medial gastrocnemius muscle, *SM* semimembranosus tendon, *arrowheads* needle. (**e**) End of the procedure; the bursa is completely drained. (**f**) Steroid injection (*asterisks*)

Parameniscal cysts: the patient is positioned according to the location of the cyst. Usually, the needle is inserted according to the major axis of the cyst. The procedure is shown in **Fig. 9.2**. When the cyst involves the superficial peroneal nerve, extreme caution should be taken to avoid the nerve fascicles. The procedure is shown in **Fig. 9.3**.

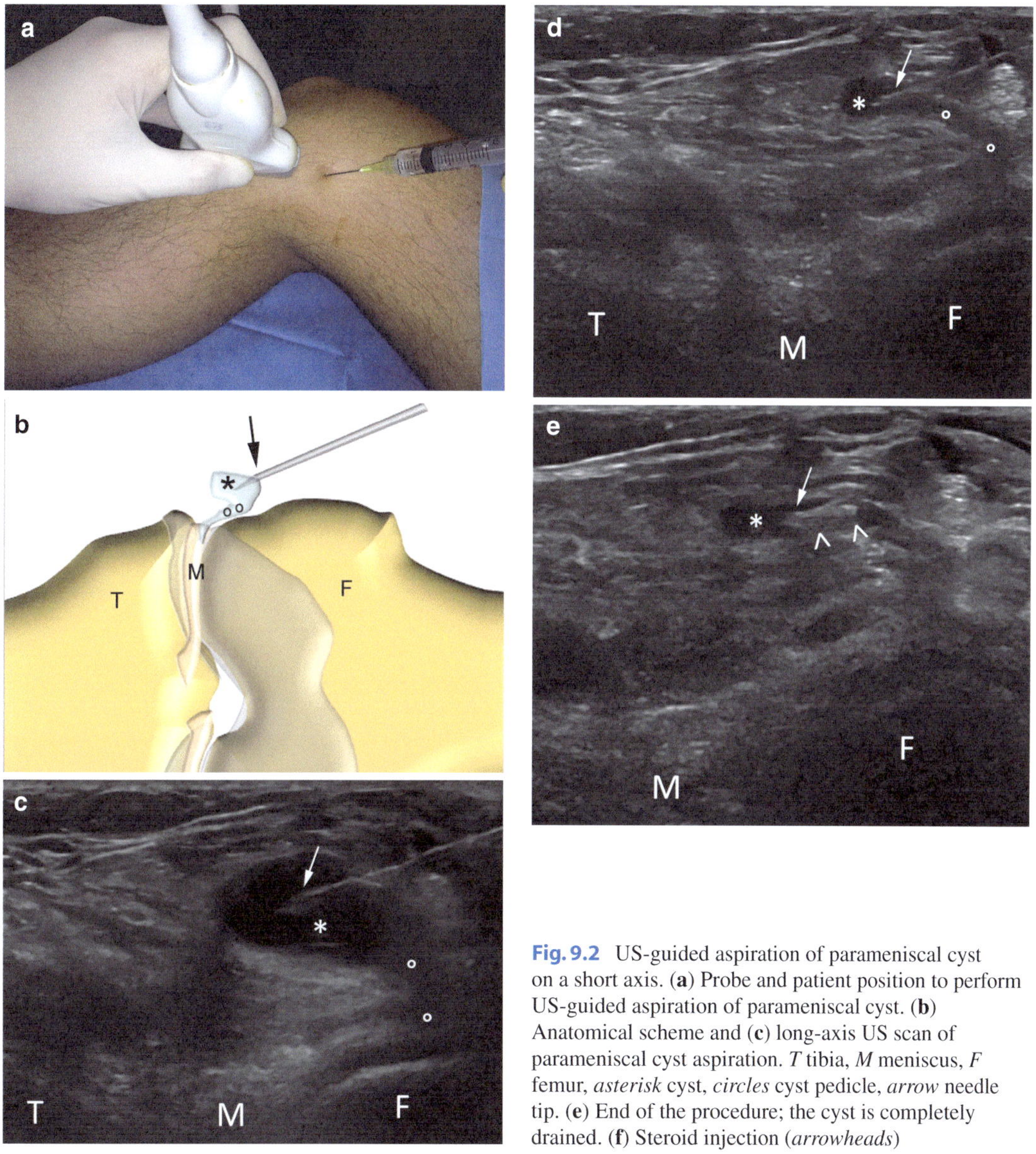

Fig. 9.2 US-guided aspiration of parameniscal cyst on a short axis. (**a**) Probe and patient position to perform US-guided aspiration of parameniscal cyst. (**b**) Anatomical scheme and (**c**) long-axis US scan of parameniscal cyst aspiration. *T* tibia, *M* meniscus, *F* femur, *asterisk* cyst, *circles* cyst pedicle, *arrow* needle tip. (**e**) End of the procedure; the cyst is completely drained. (**f**) Steroid injection (*arrowheads*)

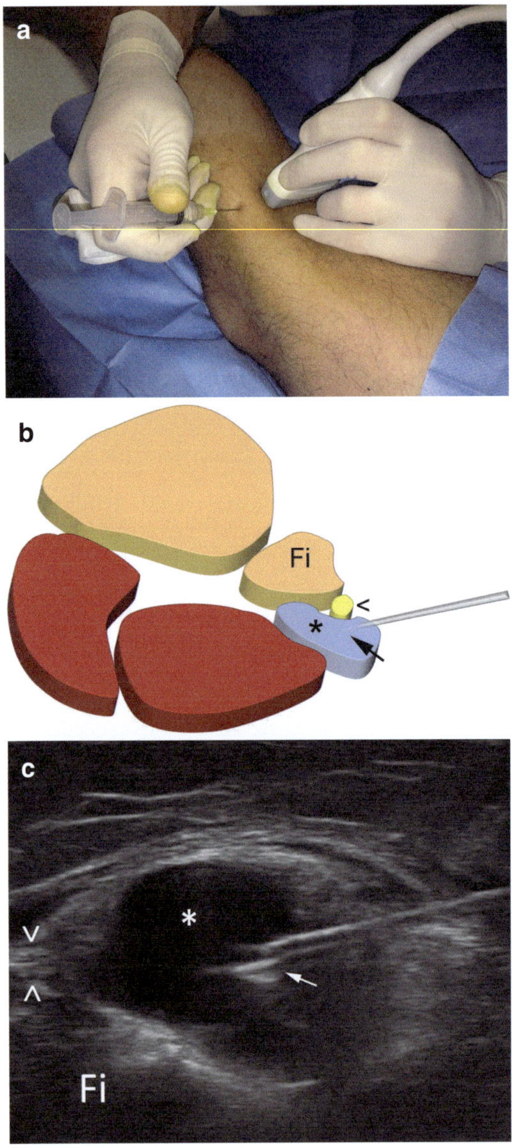

Fig. 9.3 US-guided aspiration of intraneural cyst of the superficial branch of the popliteal nerve on a short axis. (**a**) Probe and patient position to perform US-guided aspiration of intraneural cyst. (**b**) Anatomical scheme and (**c**) long-axis US scan of intraneural cyst aspiration. *Fi* fibula, *arrowheads* nerve fascicles, *arrow* needle tip, *asterisk* cyst

Goose's foot bursitis: the patient may lie on the contralateral side or prone, with the knee extended. The bursa is demonstrated either with longitudinal or sagittal scans, and the needle can be inserted with the most comfortable approach.

Prepatellar bursitis: the patient is positioned prone and the bursa is demonstrated with an axial scan over the anterior aspect of the patella. The needle is usually inserted with a lateral-medial direction.

STEP 2

A needle connected to a syringe is inserted with an in-plane approach until the needle tip enters the bursa or cyst. The content may be very dense and drainage could be extremely challenging. In these cases, the operator may inject in the bursa or in the cyst a small amount of lidocaine (5 ml) to dilute the content and aspirate it more easily. A larger shielded cannula and application of a manual compression over the bursa may also be helpful. A biopsy handle may also be used to obtain a more effective vacuum effect.

STEP 3

When the bursa or cyst is completely drained, a small amount of steroid (1 ml) is then injected, visualized with a cloudy hyperechoic appearance. This has the purpose of both reducing inflammation and helping the walls to remain collapsed. The needle is then removed, local compression is applied, and a plaster is placed over the puncture site.

Post-procedure Care

The patient is kept in observation for about 10 min. Pain after treatment may occasionally occur and it could be managed using oral NSAIDs.

Patellar Tendinopathy

10

Davide Orlandi, Francesca Lacelli,
and Giovanni Serafini

Essentials

Degenerative changes of tendons around the knee are not particularly common, with the exception of patellar tendon, as most of the forces exerted during extension are conveyed over this structure. Typically, degenerative changes are localized over the proximal insertion of the tendon on the inferior pole of the patella, where this disease is also known as "jumper's knee." However, degeneration may also occur during the tendon course. Less commonly, degeneration may occur on the distal insertion of the tendon, which is usually more prone to overload in younger subjects and develop anterior tibial apophysitis. Occasionally, overload may occur also at the distal insertion of the quadriceps tendon.

Clinical Presentation

The most common symptom is pain over the distal pole of the patella, over the proximal enthesis of the tendon. Pain is usually worsened by the execution of active movements, such as jumping or running. Swelling is not generally present.

Ultrasound Diagnosis

Ultrasound is very important for a differential diagnosis between tendinopathy and patellar chondropathy. Ultrasound shows a thickened, hypoechoic tendon, with loss of normal fibrillar echotexture. When the disease is active, power Doppler may show the presence of intense vascularization, representing angiofibroblastic proliferation. Calcifications and enthesophytes may also be present. The patellar tendon is not provided with a synovial sheath. However, a hypoechoic halo can be detected surrounding the tendon body, representing peritendinitis. Deep patellar bursitis can also be present.

Treatment Options

Conservative treatment includes rest, modification of sport activity, physical therapy, ice, and anti-inflammatory and analgesic medications. In unresponsive cases, percutaneous ultrasound-guided procedures or surgical tendinous debridement can be considered.

D. Orlandi (✉)
Department of Internal Medicine, University of Genova, Genova, Italy
e-mail: theabo@libero.it

F. Lacelli • G. Serafini
Unit of Radiology, Ospedale Santa Corona, ASL 2 Savonese, Pietra Ligure, Italy
e-mail: lafrancy78@libero.it; giovanni.serafini52@gmail.com

L.M. Sconfienza et al. (eds.), *Ultrasound-guided Musculoskeletal Procedures: The Lower Limb*, DOI 10.1007/978-88-470-5764-7_10

Interventional Procedure

Indications

Symptomatic enthesopathy of the patellar tendon

Objective

To cause local hyperemia and bleeding into the tendon, thus promoting post-procedural platelet-induced recovery phenomena

Equipment

- 1 syringe (5–10 ml)
- 20G needle
- Lidocaine (5–10 ml)
- Long-acting steroid (1 ml, 40 mg/ml)
- Plaster

How We Do It

STEP 1

The patient lies prone on the bed with the knee slightly flexed. An ultrasound scan is made to identify the proximal insertion of the tendon to plan the most comfortable approach. The needle can be inserted via a caudo-cranial or lateral-medial approach. The procedure is shown in **Fig. 10.1.**

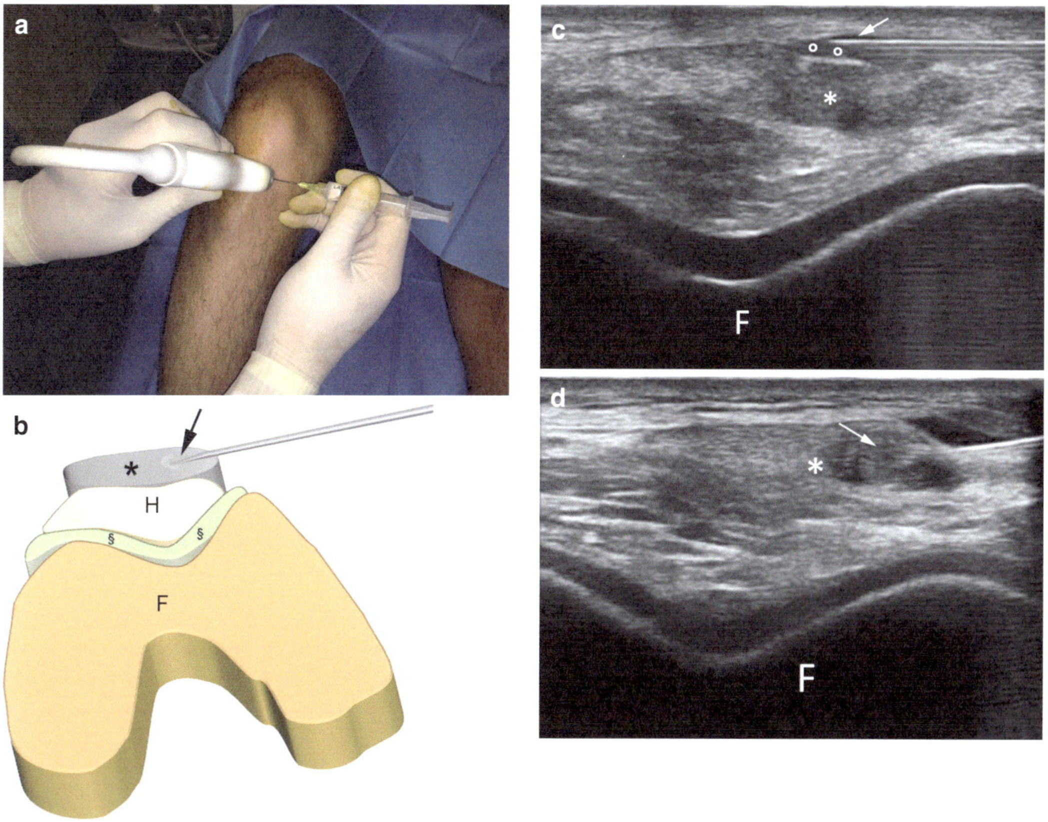

Fig. 10.1 US-guided treatment of patellar tendinopathy on a short-axis scan. (**a**) Probe and patient position to perform short-axis US-guided treatment of patellar tendinopathy. (**b**) Anatomical scheme and (**c**) US scan of patellar tendinopathy treatment, *F* femur, *§* articular cartilage, *H* Hoffa's fat pad, *asterisk* patellar tendon, *arrow* needle tip, *circles* peritendinous anesthesia. (**d**) Dry-needling procedure

STEP 2

A small amount of anesthetic is injected around the enthesis. After a couple of minutes waiting without retracting the needle, a series of 15–20 repeated punctures (dry needling) on the affected portion of the tendon is then performed. The periosteum should also be hit. Platelet-rich plasma can also be used in substitution (or in addition to) dry needling. It should be injected within the tendon fibers, in the most hypoechoic area.

STEP 3

Half-to-one mL of steroid is injected in the peritendinous soft tissues, superficially to tendon enthesis. Caution should be taken to avoid direct intratendinous injection.

At the end of the procedure, the needle is then removed and a plaster applied at the cutaneous puncture site.

Post-procedure Care

The patient is kept in observation for about 10 min. A rest period of the affected structure and associated physical therapy are suggested. Pain occurrence after treatment may occur and it could be managed using ice and oral NSAIDs.

Part III

The Ankle

11 The Ankle: Focused US Anatomy and Examination Technique

Riccardo Sartoris and Angelo Corazza

The standard US protocol includes the evaluation of four compartments of the ankle: lateral, medial, posterior, and anterior.

Lateral Compartment

The patient lies supine on the table with the knee flexed at about 90°, with the foot slightly intra-rotated.

Peroneal Tendons

The peroneal tendons should be evaluated on a short-axis scan. The evaluation must be commenced with horizontal axial scans over the proximal malleolus. At this level, the peroneal muscles and their distal myotendinous junction can be seen. Then, the probe must be moved distally following a curvilinear line that turns around the lateral malleolus tip. The peroneus brevis tendon has a typical crescent appearance and is located deep to the peroneus longus tendon, which has a typical oval shape. Long-axis scan is not useful in the evaluation of peroneal tendons, except when assessing their distal bone insertions (Fig. 11.1).

R. Sartoris (✉) • A. Corazza
Postgraduate School in Radiodiagnostics, University of Genoa, School of Medicine, Genova, Italy
e-mail: riccardo.sartoris@hotmail.it; angelcoraz@libero.it

Medial Compartment

The patient lies supine on the bed, with the knee flexed at about 90°, and the foot is slightly externally rotated.

Tarsal Tunnel

The *posterior tibial tendon*, the *flexor digitorum longus tendon*, the *tibial neurovascular bundle*, and the *flexor hallucis longus tendon* are contained in the tarsal tunnel (medial to lateral).

The tarsal tunnel can be assessed on axial scans placing one edge of the probe on the tip of the medial malleolus and the other on the Achilles tendon. The *posterior tibial tendon* must be evaluated along its whole course with axial scans, up to its main insertion on the navicular bone. This area must be assessed carefully, also with longitudinal scans, due to the complexity of the enthesis that could result in anisotropy artifacts. The presence of an accessory navicular bone is an extremely common finding. The *flexor digitorum longus* and *flexor hallucis longus tendons* must be scanned with the same approach described for the posterior tibial tendon.

The tibial neurovascular bundle can be easily seen between the posterior tibial tendon and the flexor digitorum longus tendon (Fig. 11.2).

L.M. Sconfienza et al. (eds.), *Ultrasound-guided Musculoskeletal Procedures: The Lower Limb*, DOI 10.1007/978-88-470-5764-7_11

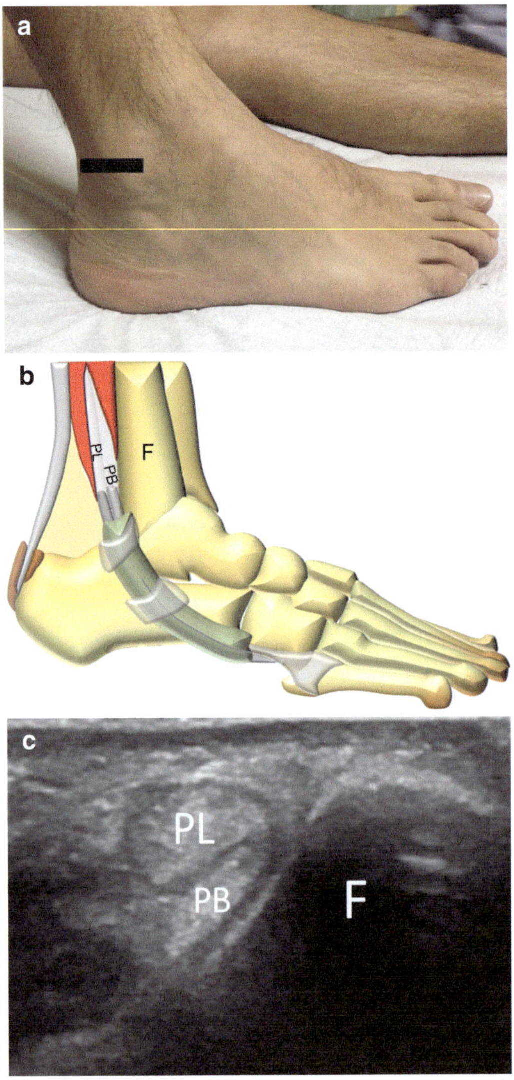

Fig. 11.1 Evaluation of the lateral ankle to assess the peroneal tendons. (**a**) The probe and patient are positioned to evaluate the peroneal tendons on a short-axis scan. (**b**) Anatomical scheme of the peroneal tendons as seen along their short axis, *F* fibula, *PL* peroneus longus, *PB* peroneus brevis. (**c**) US long-axis scan of peroneal tendons

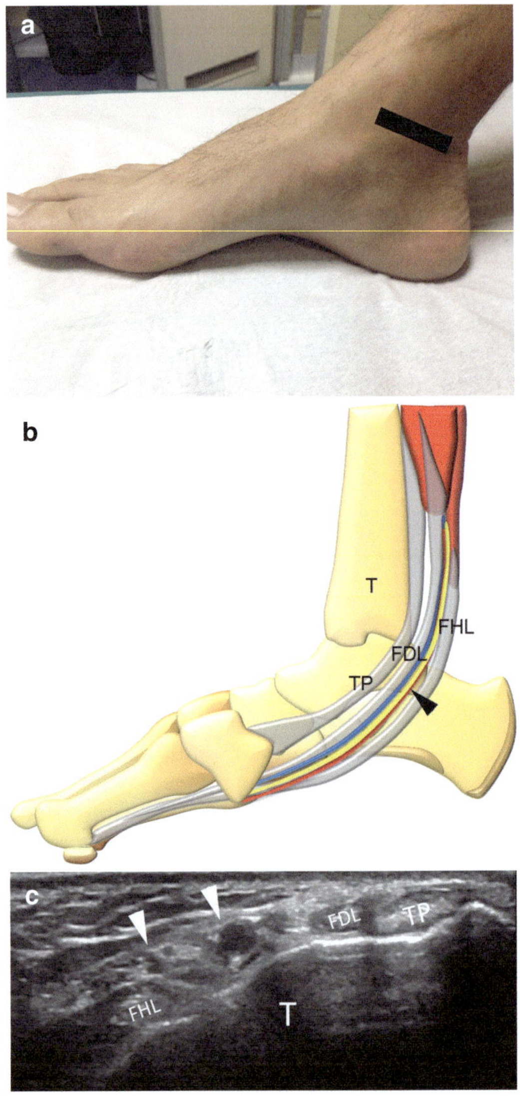

Fig. 11.2 Evaluation of the medial ankle to assess the tarsal tunnel. (**a**) The probe and patient are positioned to evaluate the tarsal tunnel on a short-axis scan. (**b**) Anatomical scheme of the tarsal tunnel as seen along their short axis, *TP* tibialis posterior tendon, *FDL* flexor digitorum longus tendon, *FHL* flexor hallucis longus tendon, *arrowheads* tibial neurovascular bundle, *T* tibia. (**c**) US long-axis scan of tarsal tunnel

Posterior Compartment

Achilles Tendon

The patient lies prone with the ankle hanging out of the bed. The Achilles tendon is assessed using both short- and long-axis scans, from the myotendinous junction to the enthesis. However, tendon thickness should be measured on short axis only.

Dynamic long-axis scans are useful to evaluate biomechanical relationships among the enthesis, the retrocalcaneal bursa, Kager's fat pad, and the posterosuperior calcaneal tubercle.

Dynamic scans in passive plantar and dorsal flexion of the ankle allow for a differential diagnosis between incomplete and complete rupture.

Posterior Tibiotalar Recess

The posterior tibiotalar recess can be assessed using coronal oblique scans on the medial side of the Achilles tendon (Fig. 11.3).

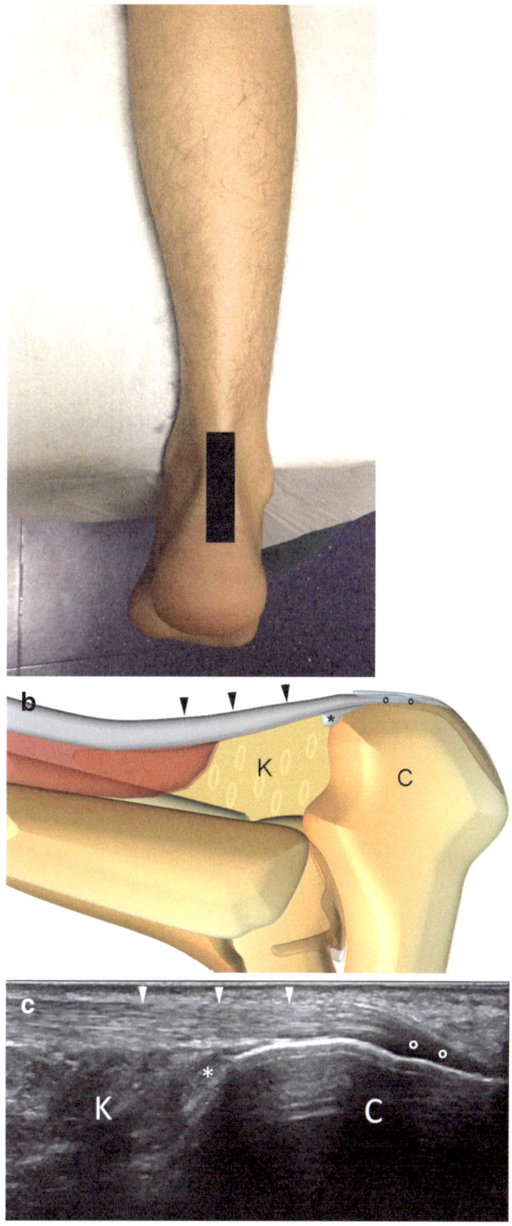

Fig. 11.3 Evaluation of the posterior ankle to assess the Achilles tendon. (**a**) The probe and patient are positioned to evaluate the Achilles tendon on a long-axis scan. (**b**) Anatomical scheme of the Achilles tendon as seen along its long axis, *C* calcaneus, *K* Kager's fat pad, *asterisk* retrocalcaneal bursa, *arrowheads* Achilles tendon, *circles* enthesis of the Achilles tendon, partially affected by anisotropy artifacts. (**c**) US long-axis scan of Achilles tendon

Anterior Compartment

The foot must placed in the same position used to assess the lateral compartment.

Anterior Tendons and Deep Peroneal Nerve

The probe must be placed on an axial plane on the anterior side of the ankle. There, the *tibialis anterior tendon*, the *extensor hallucis longus tendon*, and the *extensor digitorum longus tendon* can be seen. The tendons must be followed distally up to their insertion on the first cuneiform and on the fingers, respectively.

The *deep peroneal neurovascular bundle* can be seen deeply between the extensor hallucis longus and the extensor digitorum longus tendons.

Anterior Tibiotalar Recess

The anterior tibiotalar recess can be assessed performing a longitudinal scan on the anterior aspect of the ankle, between the extensor tendons.

The anterior tibiotalar recess appears like a triangular hyperechoic area, when not distended by fluid. A thin layer of cartilage of the talus can be also seen (Fig. 11.4).

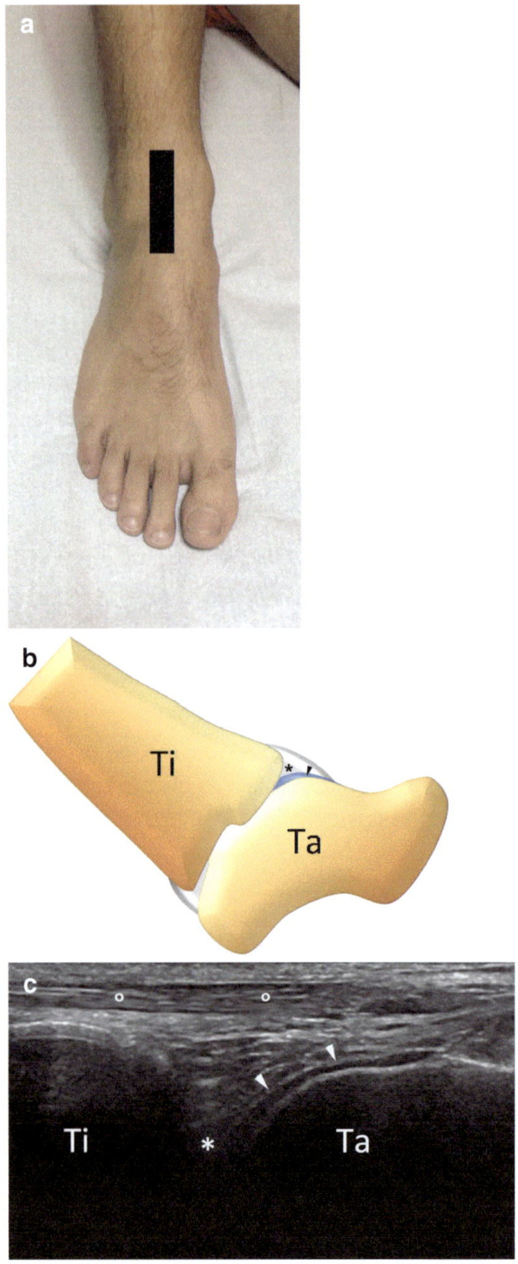

Fig. 11.4 Evaluation of the anterior ankle to assess the anterior tibiotalar recess. (**a**) The probe and patient are positioned to evaluate the anterior tibiotalar recess on a long-axis scan. (**b**) Anatomical scheme of the anterior tibiotalar recess as seen along its long axis, *Ti* tibia, *Ta* talus, *arrowheads* cartilage, *asterisk* joint space, *circles* overlying extensor hallucis longus tendon. (**c**) US long-axis scan of Achilles tendon

Ankle Intra-articular Injections

12

Angelo Corazza and Riccardo Sartoris

Essentials

Intra-articular injections of the ankle can be performed to treat a variety of pathological conditions. The drugs administered in these cases may be anti-inflammatory agents, such as steroids that may be indicated for patients with ankle osteoarthritis (OA) refractory to non-pharmacologic or analgesic and NSAIDs therapy or viscosupplements, such as hyaluronic acid, which are injected to decelerate the physiological process of OA. Analgesic drugs can be injected for diagnostic purposes in the differential diagnosis between intra- and extra-articular pathology.

Clinical Presentation

Patients affected with primary OA are often >55 years old and overweight. Secondary OA develops in younger individuals with a story of trauma, tarsal coalescence, or flatfoot. The main symptom is pain and joint stiffness, variably associated with swelling or tenderness in the ankle joint and inability to flex the ankle to perform routine activities such as moderate walking. Sometimes, a sound or feeling of bone rubbing against bone is reported.

A. Corazza (✉) • R. Sartoris
Postgraduate School in Radiodiagnostics, University of Genova, School of Medicine, Genova, Italy
e-mail: angelcoraz@libero.it; riccardo.sartoris@hotmail.it

Ultrasound Diagnosis

The diagnosis of ankle OA requires plain film examination. However, US can demonstrate the presence of joint effusion, synovial hypertrophy, and presence of osteophytes.

Treatment Options

Conservative treatment includes weight loss, physical therapy, anti-inflammatory and analgesic medications, and intra-articular injections of steroids or hyaluronates. At later stage, ankle joint replacement can be performed.

Interventional Procedure

Objective

To deliver anti-inflammatory, analgesic, or viscosupplement drugs within the joint space

Equipment

- 1 syringe (2–5 ml)
- 20G needle
- Long-acting steroid (1 ml, 40 mg/ml) or hyaluronic acid (2–4 ml)
- Plaster

L.M. Sconfienza et al. (eds.), *Ultrasound-guided Musculoskeletal Procedures: The Lower Limb*, DOI 10.1007/978-88-470-5764-7_12

How We Do It

Intra-articular injection at the level of the ankle is generally performed with palpation guidance in the anterolateral recess. However, the presence of articular osteophytes could reduce the success rate of this procedure. Particular caution should be taken to avoid the anterior neurovascular bundle. Out-plane approach can be used, though suffering from a more difficult visualization of the needle tip. Lateral (in-plane) approach allows for a direct and continuous visualization of the needle along the whole path in soft tissues, though it can be limited by the presence of anterior tendons and neurovascular bundle.

The patient lies in supine position, with the lower limb slightly intra-rotated (about 15–20°). The location of the neurovascular bundle should be double-checked to avoid accidental punctures. Then, the probe is rotated 90°. A correct scanning plane should demonstrate the tibial distal epiphysis, the talus covered by hyaline cartilage and the joint recess.

Caudo-Cranial Approach

STEP 1

With the articular joint space centered in the middle of the screen, the 20G needle is connected to the syringe filled with anesthetic and inserted laterally to the distal side of the probe with a caudal-cranial direction. Small cutaneous anesthesia is made and the needle is advanced. Generally, the angle of needle insertion ranges around 30°. With this approach, the whole path of the needle can be visualized in real time, and slight corrections of the direction can be made. Once the joint space is reached, a small amount of anesthetic can be injected to confirm the correct intra-articular positioning of the needle tip. There should be no resistance to the injection; if this is not the case, a short retraction (1–2 mm) of the needle should be considered, as the needle tip may be pointed against the tibia or the talus.

STEP 2

The intra-articular injection should determine a distension of the joint recess according to the amount of fluid injected. Note that steroid solution has a hypoechoic appearance with many hyperechoic dots inside, while hyaluronic acid is highly echogenic. At the end of the injection, the needle can be removed and a plaster is applied at the cutaneous site of approach.

Coaxial Approach

The articular joint space is centered on the screen, and a 20G spinal needle is inserted vertically at the level of the middle to the probe, with a very slight lateral-to-medial angulation (about 5°) to reach the joint space visualized in the scanning plane. Along its path, the needle tip is visualized indirectly, by means of slight movements of superficial soft tissues; when the intra-articular position is reached, it is visualized as a hyperechoic dot in the articular recess. An intra-articular injection of a small amount (1–2 cc) of local anesthetic can help in confirming the correct position of the needle tip.

Post-procedural Care

The patient should be kept under observation for at least 15 min after the procedure. Pain may occur after treatment and is managed with oral NSAIDs (Fig. 12.1).

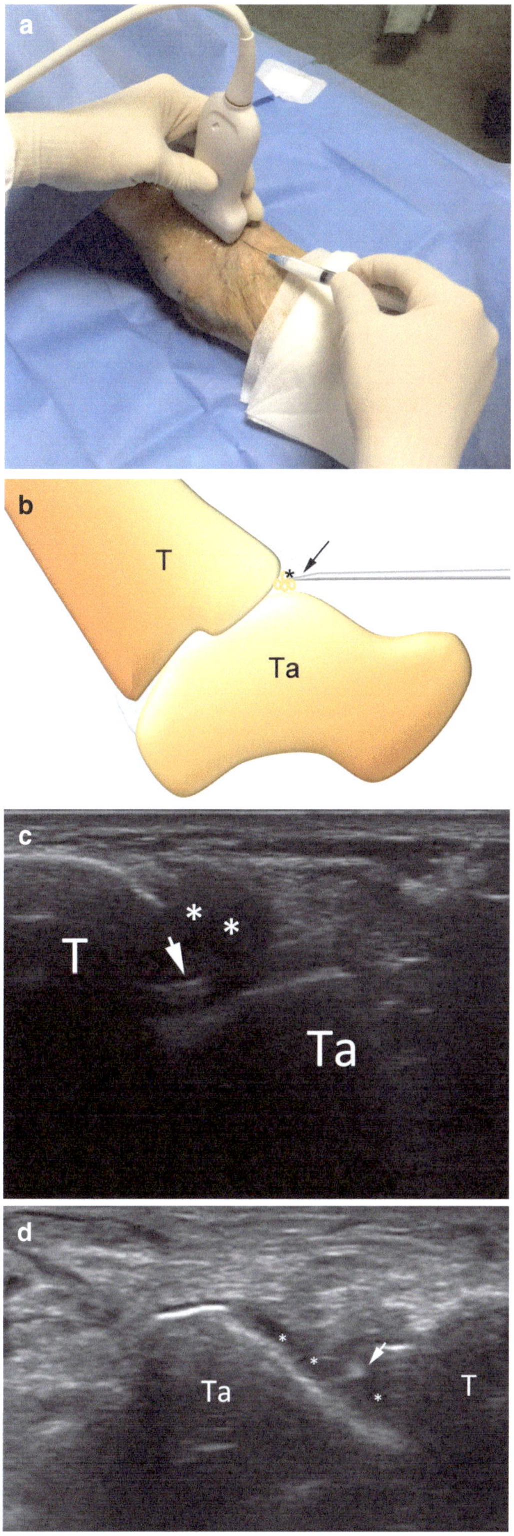

Fig. 12.1 US-guided intra-articular ankle injection. (**a**) Probe and patient position to perform long-axis US-guided intra-articular ankle injection. (**b**) Anatomical scheme and (**c**) US scan of long-axis intra-articular ankle injection, *T* tibia, *Ta* talus, *asterisk* articular fluid, *arrow* needle. (**d**) US scan of intra-articular ankle injection with coaxial approach

13 Achilles Tendinopathy

Davide Orlandi and Enzo Silvestri

Essentials

Achilles tendinopathy is a degenerative tendinous disorder that commonly involves the hypovascular area located from 2 to 6 cm above the calcaneal insertion. It is commonly considered the result of multiple micro-tears that do not heal because of poor tendon vascularity. Achilles tendinopathy is a common condition in the adult population. In 59 % of patients, it is related to sports activities, and 53 % of them are runners. Some intrinsic factors (e.g., gender, age, and overweight) and extrinsic factors (e.g., functional overload, poor footwear, and training errors) play an important role in the development of chronic tendinopathy. Achilles tendinopathy is characterized by degenerative changes that could be located along the tendon course or at the enthesis. Histological features in the early stages of the disease are focal areas of asymptomatic intratendineous damage without signs of inflammation. Histological appearance of degenerative damage begins and progresses long before onset of symptoms. This delay causes late therapeutic approaches to be less successful.

D. Orlandi (✉)
Department of Internal Medicine, University of Genova, Genova, Italy
e-mail: theabo@libero.it

E. Silvestri
Unit of Radiology, Ospedale Evangelico Internazionale, Genova, Italy
e-mail: silvi.enzo@gmail.com

Treatment Options

First-line therapy usually consists of ice application, immobility, and NSAIDs. Shockwave therapy can reduce symptoms in the middle term. Surgical debridement is reserved for refractory cases. US-guided scarification (dry needling) can be considered as a minimally invasive option. New theories of tendon regeneration have been focused on the role of platelets and the development of different therapeutic strategies in the treatment of chronic tendinopathy. Platelets participate in the healing process by removing necrotic tissues and stimulating regeneration and healing of the tissues.

Indications

Peritendinitis without signs of tendon degeneration

- Simple steroid injection in the peritoneum
- Hydrodilatation (injection of 30–40 ml of a saline and local anesthetic solution in the peritoneum)

L.M. Sconfienza et al. (eds.), *Ultrasound-guided Musculoskeletal Procedures: The Lower Limb*, DOI 10.1007/978-88-470-5764-7_13

Insertional and pre-insertional overload tendinopathy of the Achilles tendon

- Dry-needling and steroid injection
- Dry-needling + autologous blood injection and steroid injection
- Dry-needling + platelet-rich plasma injection

Note that dry-needling procedures are contraindicated in case of traumatic lesions of the Achilles tendon.

Equipment

- 1 syringe (5–10 ml)
- 1 syringe (1–2 ml)
- 20G needle
- Lidocaine (5–10 ml)
- Long-acting steroid (1 ml, 40 mg/ml)
- Plaster

Objective

To cause local hyperemia and bleeding into the tendon, thus promoting post-procedural platelets-induced recovery phenomena

How We Do It

The patient lies prone with the foot hanging outside the examination bed.

The Achilles tendon is visualized with longitudinal US scan. The proximal portion of the probe is placed on the hyperechoic bony line of the calcaneus, while the distal part of the probe is aligned according to the Achilles tendon. Then, the probe should be moved to detect the most affected site. Rotate the probe 90° to evaluate tendon on its short axis.

Longitudinal Approach

The 20G needle is inserted with an in-plane approach in a distal-proximal direction Figs. 13.1. Anesthetic is injected along the path of the needle, in the peritendinous soft tissues, and in the degenerated portions of the tendon. Then perform a series of 15–20 repeated punctures (dry needling) on the most degenerate portion of the tendon to obtain a mild bleeding. At this point, a small amount of autologous blood or platelet-rich plasma can be injected inside the tendon fibers to enhance the effects of the procedure.

Complete the procedure retracting the needle outside the tendon and injecting 1 ml of steroid into the peritendinous soft tissues, superficially to the tendon enthesis. The needle is then removed and a plaster applied.

Lateral Approach

The 20G needle is inserted with an in-plane approach in a medial to lateral direction Figs. 13.2. With this approach, it is easier to detect small degenerative changes inside the tendon and to treat them selectively.

The dry-needling procedure is performed as above.

Post-procedural Care

The patient is kept under observation for about 10 min. Pain may occur after treatment and can be managed with oral NSAIDs.

Patients are advised to use an orthotic support and to reduce their overload activity, although no systematic rest period is suggested.

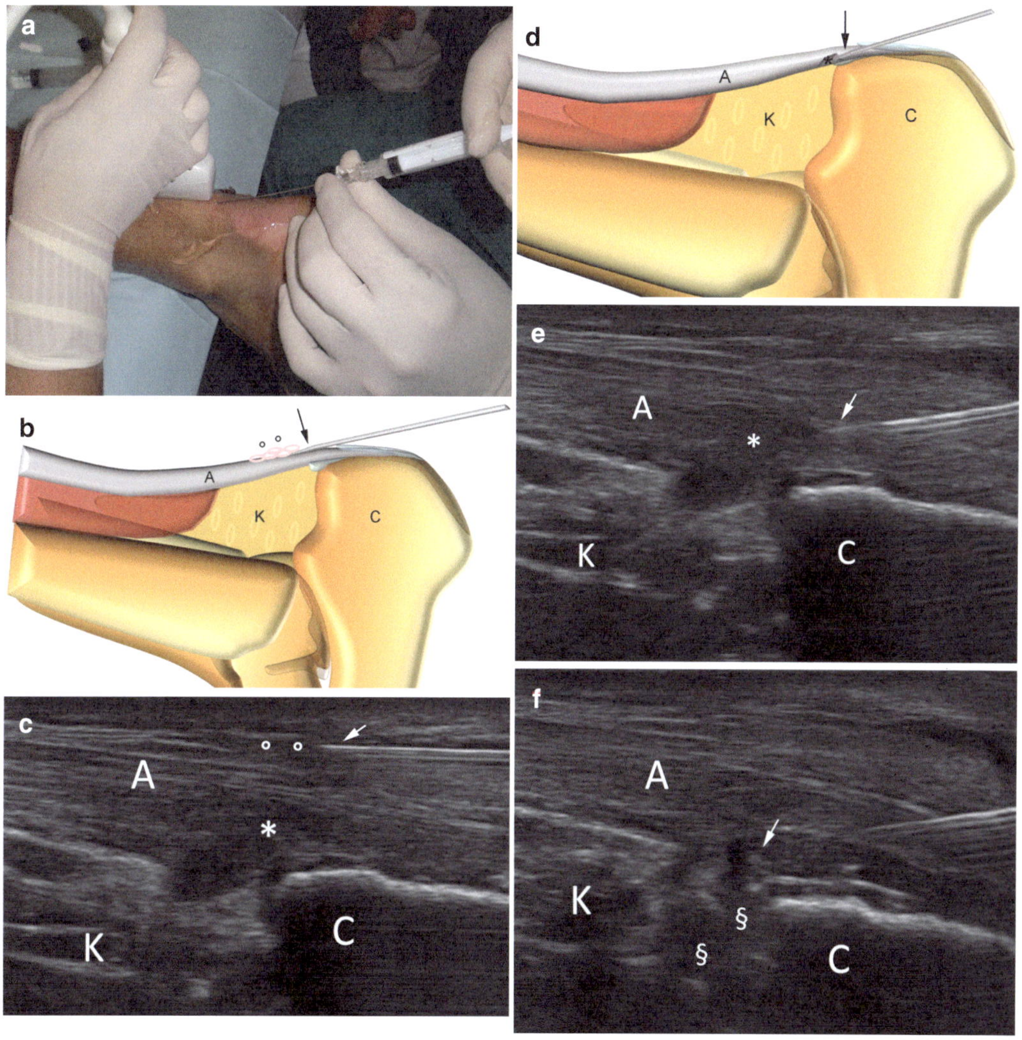

Fig. 13.1 US-guided treatment of Achilles tendinopathy on a long-axis scan. (**a**) Probe and patient position to perform long-axis US-guided treatment of Achilles tendinopathy. (**b**) Anatomical scheme and (**c**) US scan of peritendinous anesthetic injection, *A* Achilles tendon, *C* calcaneus, *K* Kager's triangle, *arrow* needle tip, *circle* anesthetic, *asterisk* intratendinous degenerated area. (**d**) Anatomical scheme and (**e**) dry-needling procedure. (**f**) Steroid injection in the retrocalcaneal bursa (*§*)

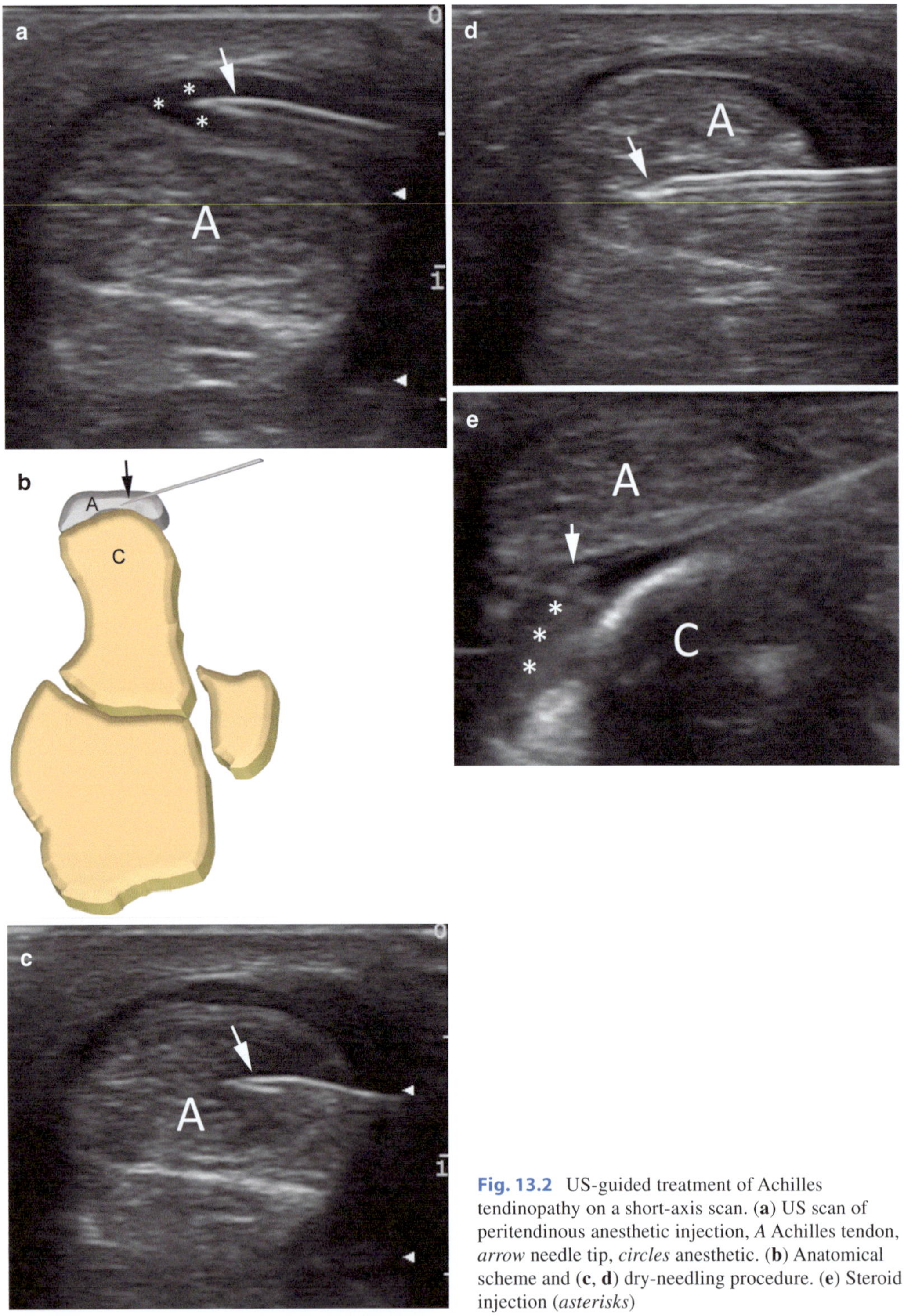

Fig. 13.2 US-guided treatment of Achilles tendinopathy on a short-axis scan. (**a**) US scan of peritendinous anesthetic injection, *A* Achilles tendon, *arrow* needle tip, *circles* anesthetic. (**b**) Anatomical scheme and (**c**, **d**) dry-needling procedure. (**e**) Steroid injection (*asterisks*)

14 Drainage of Articular Ganglia Around the Ankle

Emanuele Fabbro and Giulio Ferrero

Essentials

Ganglion cysts are the most common benign soft-tissue lesions of the ankle. They predominantly occur in young adults. In 60–70 % of cases, the ganglion cyst originates from the subtalar joint and communicates with the synovial joint via a pedicle. In 20 % of the cases, ganglia are found on the anterior aspect of the ankle, arising from the tibiotalar joint or from the talonavicular joint.

Etiology

Ganglia are articular cysts that originate from the articular cavity. The exact mechanism of ganglion formation remains unknown.

Clinical Presentation

On examination, subtalar joint ganglia are usually 2–5-cm lumps, rarely accompanied by signs of inflammation.

While ganglia are frequently asymptomatic, symptoms may include numbness or ankle pain, especially during activities; functional limitation; or a decrease in strength. In some cases, subtalar joint ganglia may cause tarsal tunnel syndrome by compressing the posterior tibial nerve or its branches within the tarsal tunnel.

Ultrasound Diagnosis

Subtalar joint ganglia have a typical cystic pattern on US, i.e., roundish or oval hypo/anechoic appearance, well delimited by a thin and regular wall. When the cyst content is not exactly hypo/anechoic, differentiating a ganglia from other pathological conditions could be challenging.

Treatment Options

Typically, ganglion cysts may reduce spontaneously their size, as jelly content may resorpt through the joint space. US-guided drainage could be performed but a recurrence rate up to 30 % has been described. Surgical excision represents the standard of care in this condition, although recurrence is not uncommon.

E. Fabbro (✉) • G. Ferrero
Unit of Radiology, Ospedale Santa Corona, ASL 2 Savonese, Pietra Ligure, Italy
e-mail: emanuele.fabbro@gmail.com; giulio.ferrero@gmail.com

L.M. Sconfienza et al. (eds.), *Ultrasound-guided Musculoskeletal Procedures: The Lower Limb*, DOI 10.1007/978-88-470-5764-7_14

Interventional Procedure

Indications

Diagnostic aspiration or therapeutic pain relief. Intra-gangliar injection of steroids

Objective

To drain the articular ganglion and deliver steroid within the joint space

Equipment

- 1 syringe (5–10 ml)
- 16–20 G needle
- Lidocaine (5 ml)
- Long-acting steroid (1 ml, 40 mg/ml)
- Plaster

How We Do It

STEP 1

US evaluation should be performed with the patient lying prone with the legs extended and the feet projecting over the examination table end. The subtalar join ganglion is demonstrated by a proximal to distal, lateral to medial oblique scan performed few millimeters above the fibular head. The needle is inserted with an in-plane cranio-caudal approach to reach the ganglion space (**Fig. 14.1**).

STEP 2

A needle connected to a syringe is inserted with an in-plane approach until the needle tip enters the ganglion walls. Usually, the ganglion content is very dense and drainage could be extremely challenging. In these cases, the use of a larger needle and a biopsy handle may also be used to obtain a more effective vacuum effect.

STEP 3

When the ganglion is completely drained, a small amount of steroid (1 ml) and local anesthetic is then injected. The needle is then removed and a plaster applied at the cutaneous puncture site.

Post-procedure Care

The patient is kept in observation for about 10 min. Pain occurrence after treatment may occasionally occur and it could be managed using oral NSAIDs.

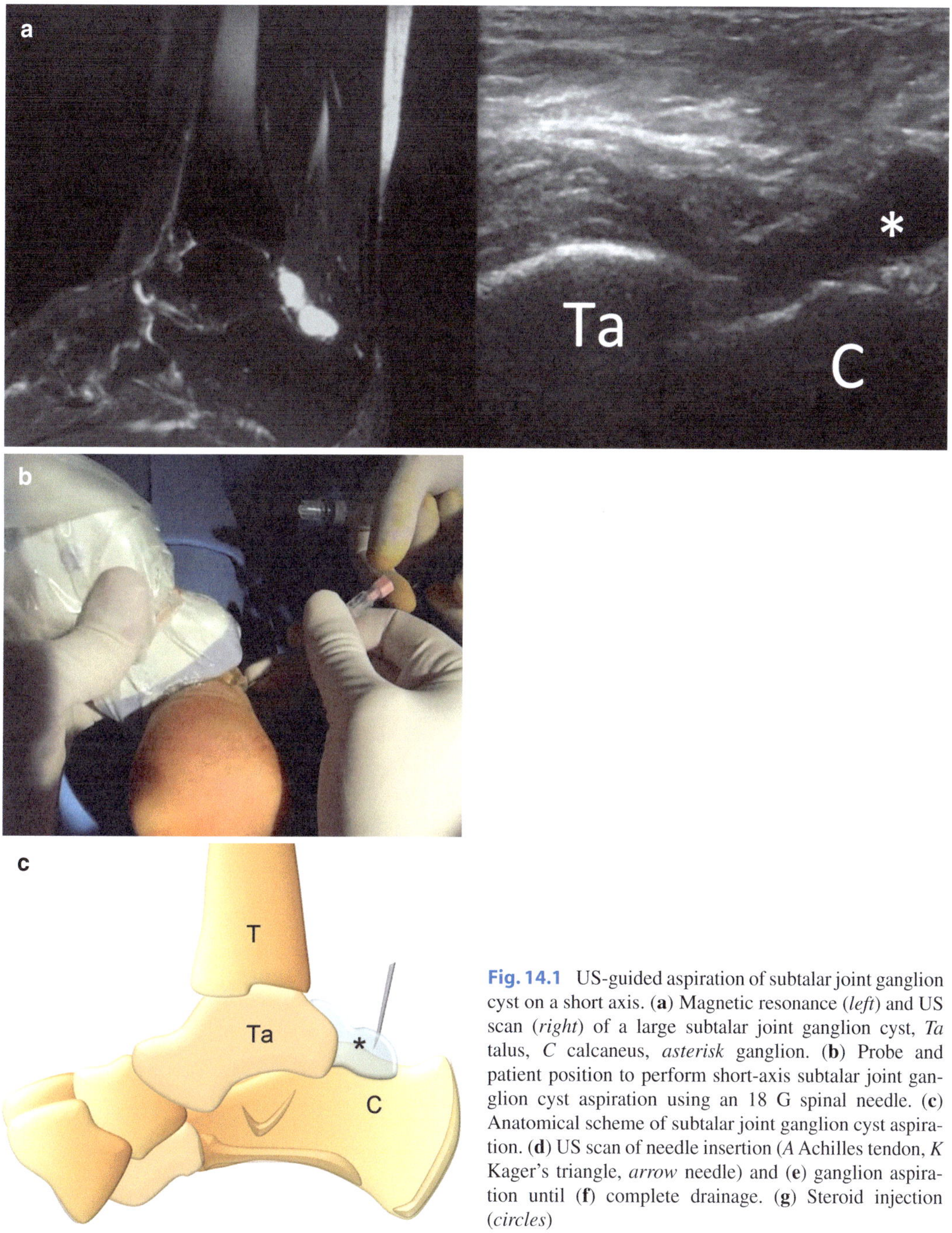

Fig. 14.1 US-guided aspiration of subtalar joint ganglion cyst on a short axis. (**a**) Magnetic resonance (*left*) and US scan (*right*) of a large subtalar joint ganglion cyst, *Ta* talus, *C* calcaneus, *asterisk* ganglion. (**b**) Probe and patient position to perform short-axis subtalar joint ganglion cyst aspiration using an 18 G spinal needle. (**c**) Anatomical scheme of subtalar joint ganglion cyst aspiration. (**d**) US scan of needle insertion (*A* Achilles tendon, *K* Kager's triangle, *arrow* needle) and (**e**) ganglion aspiration until (**f**) complete drainage. (**g**) Steroid injection (*circles*)

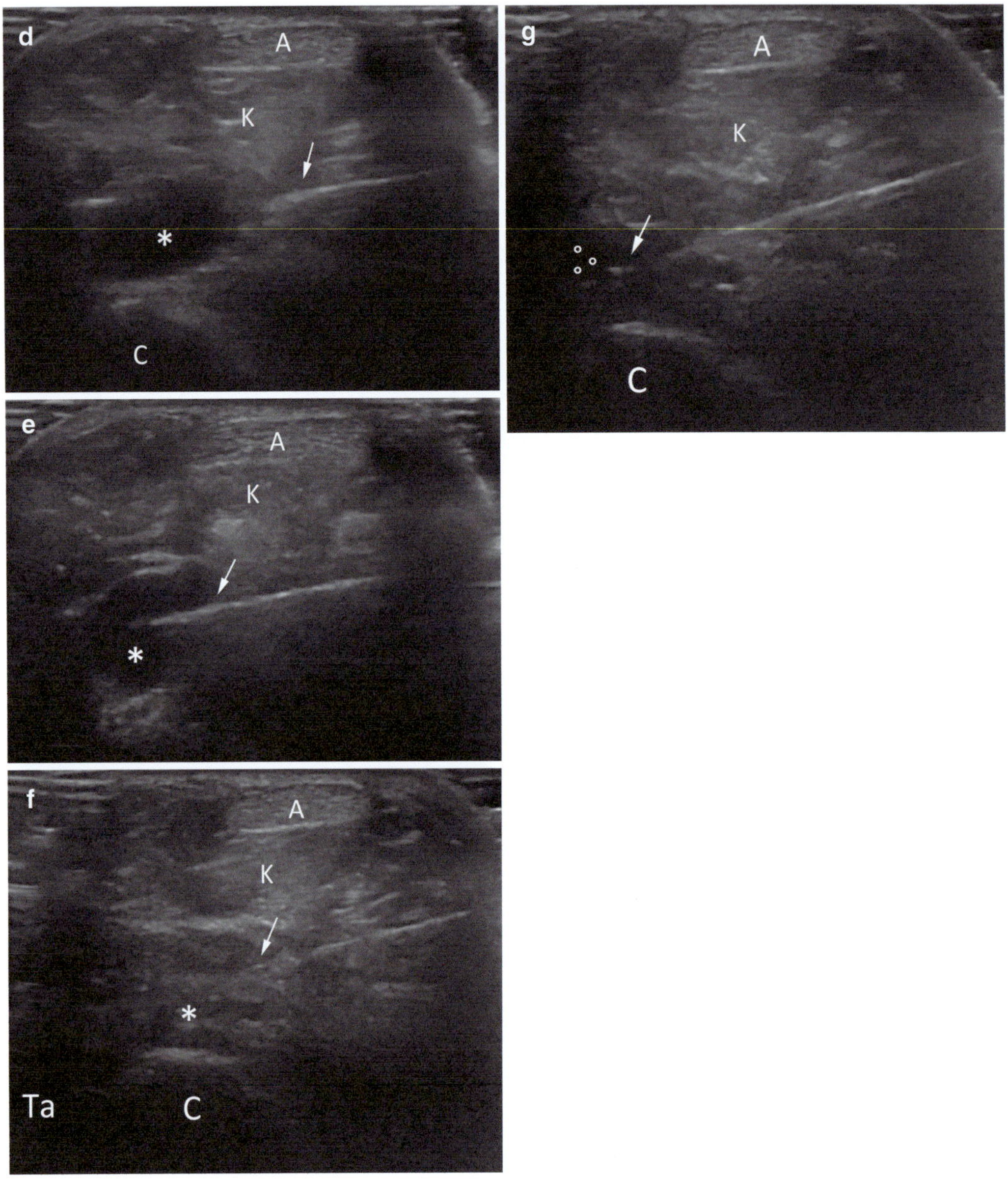

Fig. 14.1 (continued)

Deep Retrocalcaneal Bursa Injection

15

Angelo Corazza and Silvia Perugin Bernardi

Essentials

Deep retrocalcaneal bursa is a synovial bursa located deep to the Achilles tendon acting as friction attenuator between the Achilles tendon and the posterior superior aspect of the calcaneus. This structure allows for a smooth gliding between these structures during ankle movements, and in normal conditions, it cannot be demonstrated as it contains only a small amount of fluid.

Deep retrocalcaneal bursitis is frequently a sport-related overuse syndrome reflecting an overload of the hindfoot, although it is also reported as an isolated primary pathology. Also, deep retrocalcaneal bursitis could be associated with inflammatory or degenerative ankle conditions.

Clinical Presentation

When distension and inflammation of the deep retrocalcaneal bursa are present, symptoms can worsen with pressure of the probe and can vary with active and passive ankle flexion.

Prolonged runs on hard surfaces, repetitive sport movements stressing the bursa through the Achilles tendon, and the presence of a hypertrophic posterosuperior calcaneal tubercle (e.g., Haglund deformity) are the main causes which lead to repetitive microtraumas and consequent inflammation of the deep retrocalcaneal bursa.

Ultrasound Diagnosis

Ultrasound can easily detect distension of the deep retrocalcaneal bursa, demonstrating a well-defined anechoic fluid collection between Achilles tendon and the superficial aspect of the calcaneus. If fluid distension is not clearly detectable, dynamic long-axis scan with flexion and extension of the ankle allows for squeezing bursal fluid. It also allows for evaluating biomechanical relationships among the enthesis, the retrocalcaneal bursa, Kager's fat pad, and the posterosuperior calcaneal tubercle.

Bursal walls can thicken in chronic cases, or internal echogenicity can be present in rheumatic patients due to the presence of a synovial hypertrophy.

Treatment Options

Conservative treatment includes rest, weight loss, physical therapy, ice, and NSAIDs and analgesic medications. US-guided aspiration and subsequent steroid injection are recommended in the case of large bursa. Surgery may be required

A. Corazza (✉) • S.P. Bernardi
Postgraduate School in Radiodiagnostics, University of Genova, School of Medicine, Genova, Italy
e-mail: angelcoraz@libero.it; silvy-86-@hotmail.it

L.M. Sconfienza et al. (eds.), *Ultrasound-guided Musculoskeletal Procedures: The Lower Limb*, DOI 10.1007/978-88-470-5764-7_15

to treat any possible underlying conditions (e.g., Haglund deformity).

Interventional Procedure

Indications

Diagnostic aspiration or therapeutic pain relief. Intra-bursal injection of steroids. Contraindicated if suspected or known bursal infection or in the presence of overlying cellulitis or infection and hypersensitivity to corticosteroids

Objective

To deliver anti-inflammatory drugs within the affected bursal space

Equipment

- 1 syringe (5 ml)
- 23G needle
- Lidocaine (1 ml)
- Long-acting steroid (1 ml, 40 mg/ml)
- Plaster

How We Do It

STEP 1

US evaluation must be performed with the patient lying prone with the legs extended and the feet hanging over the table end. The deep retrocalcaneal bursa is first demonstrated by a longitudinal scan performed on the long axis of the Achilles tendon. Then the probe is rotated by 90° and a short-axis scan is performed. The needle is then inserted with an in-plane lateral to medial approach under the Achilles tendon to reach the bursal space (**Fig. 15.1**).

STEP 2

When the needle tip is inserted inside the bursa, a small amount of steroid (1 ml) and local anesthetic (1 ml) is then injected in the bursa. The needle is then removed and a plaster applied at the cutaneous puncture site.

Post-procedure Care

The patient is kept in observation for about 10 min. Pain occurrence after treatment may occasionally occur and it could be managed using oral NSAIDs.

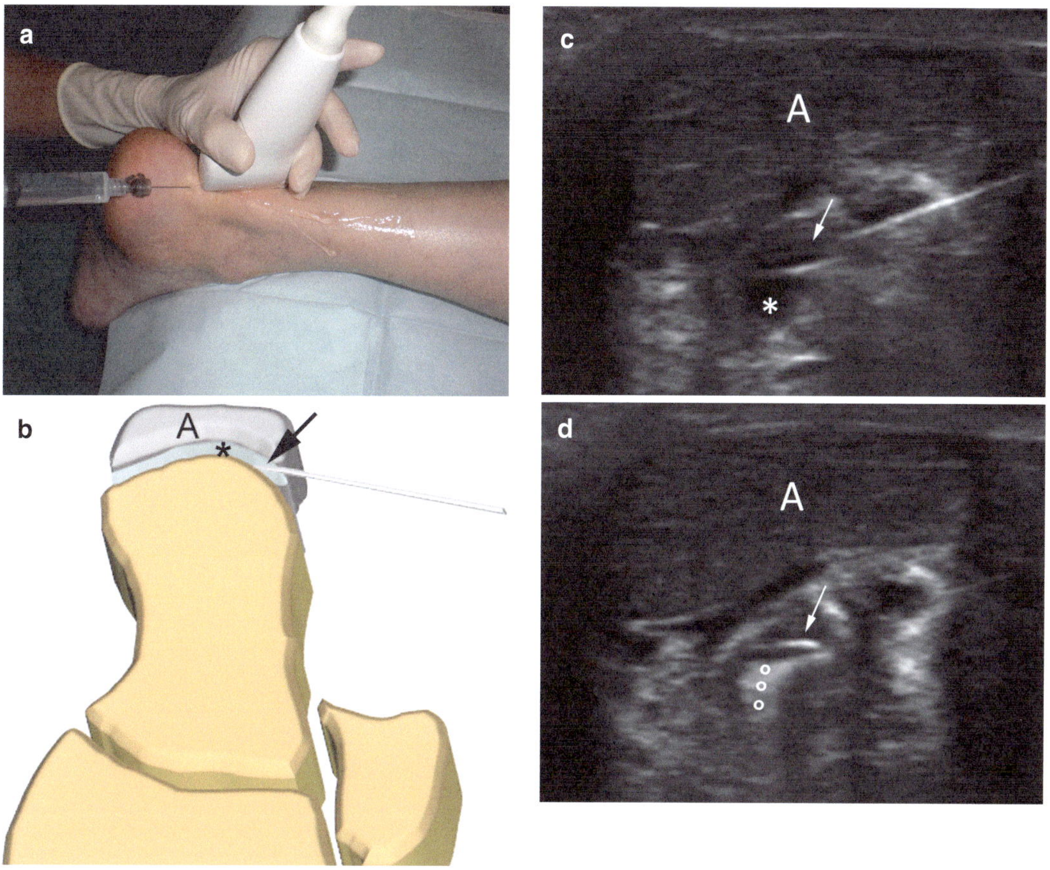

Fig. 15.1 US-guided treatment of deep retrocalcaneal bursitis on a short oblique axis. (**a**) Probe and patient position to perform US-guided treatment of deep retrocalcaneal bursitis. (**b**) Anatomical scheme and (**c**) US image of needle insertion within a distended bursa, *A* Achilles tendon, *arrow* needle, *asterisk* distended bursa. (**d**) Steroid injection (*circles*)

16 Treatment of Flexor and Extensor Tendon Sheath Tenosynovitis

Riccardo Sartoris and Alice Arcidiacono

Essentials

Ankle tendons provided by a synovial sheath (e.g., peroneal, tibialis posterior tendons) can be affected by acute or chronic tenosynovitis, which can cause pain and functional limitations. Acute tenosynovitis is characterized by fluid effusion within the tendon sheath, while chronic tenosynovitis usually presents with synovial thickening or proliferation. The lateral compartment differs from the others, as, in case of calcaneofibular ligament tear, there could be a communication between joint space and synovial sheath. In this case, sheath effusion frequently occurs in conjunction with joint effusion and should not be treated alone. Even in these cases, steroid injection is a valid option, as it is able to reduce pain and effusion. Sometimes, hyaluronic acid may be injected to improve tendon sliding and to stretch a retinaculum.

Interventional Procedure

Indications

If the condition is symptomatic and limits daily life activities, then US-guided percutaneous treatment is indicated. There are no specific contraindications to this procedure.

Objective

Early or subacute tenosynovitis responds well to corticosteroid injection, with the anti-inflammatory effects possibly resulting in relief from both pain and swelling. Advanced disease stages, characterized by a severe stenosis of the compartment due to retinaculum thickening, may benefit from a first injection of steroid, followed by 1–2 weeks delayed hyaluronic acid injection. This second step has the advantage of both improving tendon sliding and stretching the thickened retinaculum.

Note that such affections may occur when congenital or acquired flatfoot or hindfoot deformity are present.

Equipment

- 25G or smaller needle
- 1 syringe (1–2 ml)
- Long-acting steroid (1 ml, 40 mg/ml)
- Low-molecular-weight hyaluronic acid (2 ml, optional)
- Plaster

R. Sartoris (✉) • A. Arcidiacono
Postgraduate School in Radiodiagnostics,
University of Genoa, School of Medicine,
Genova, Italy
e-mail: riccardo.sartoris@hotmail.it;
alice.arcidiacono@hotmail.com

L.M. Sconfienza et al. (eds.), *Ultrasound-guided Musculoskeletal Procedures: The Lower Limb*, DOI 10.1007/978-88-470-5764-7_16

How We Do It

STEP 1

The patient is positioned in a different way according to the tendon to treat (see below). A US scan is made to identify the tendon course and to assess the most comfortable percutaneous approach.

Peroneal Tendons

US evaluation must be performed with the patient lying prone with the legs extended and the feet projecting over the examination table end.

Peroneal tendons are first demonstrated by an axial scan performed on the lateral compartment of the ankle, just above and posteriorly to the fibular head. Then the US probe is swiped down following the tendon course on their short axis in order to find where the sheath effusion is more relevant.

Flexor Tendons

US evaluation must be performed with the patient lying prone with the legs extended and the feet projecting over the examination table end.

Flexor tendons are first demonstrated by an axial scan performed on the medial compartment of the ankle, just above and posteriorly to the tibial head. Then the US probe is swiped down following the tendon course on their short axis in order to find where the sheath effusion is more relevant.

Extensor Tendons

US evaluation must be performed with the patient lying supine with the legs extended and the heels placed on the examination table.

Extensor tendons are first demonstrated by the same longitudinal scan on the anterior side of the ankle performed for the evaluation of the tibiotalar joint. Then the US probe is rotated by 90° in order to detect the extensor tendons on their short axis. Then the US probe is swiped up and down following the tendon course on their short axis in order to find where effusion is more relevant.

STEP 2

We prefer to use a short-axis lateral approach to treat ankle tenosynovitis, as with this approach accidental intratendinous injections can be easily avoided. When the sheath effusion is detected, the needle is inserted within the tendon sheath and the drug is injected.

Longitudinal Approach

Note that a long-axis approach is also possible. With this approach, the needle is carefully inserted within the tendon sheath on its long axis.

Post-procedural Care

The patient is kept under observation for about 10 min. Pain may occur after treatment and is managed with oral NSAIDs. Patients are advised to reduce their manual activity, although no systematic rest period is suggested (Fig. 16.1).

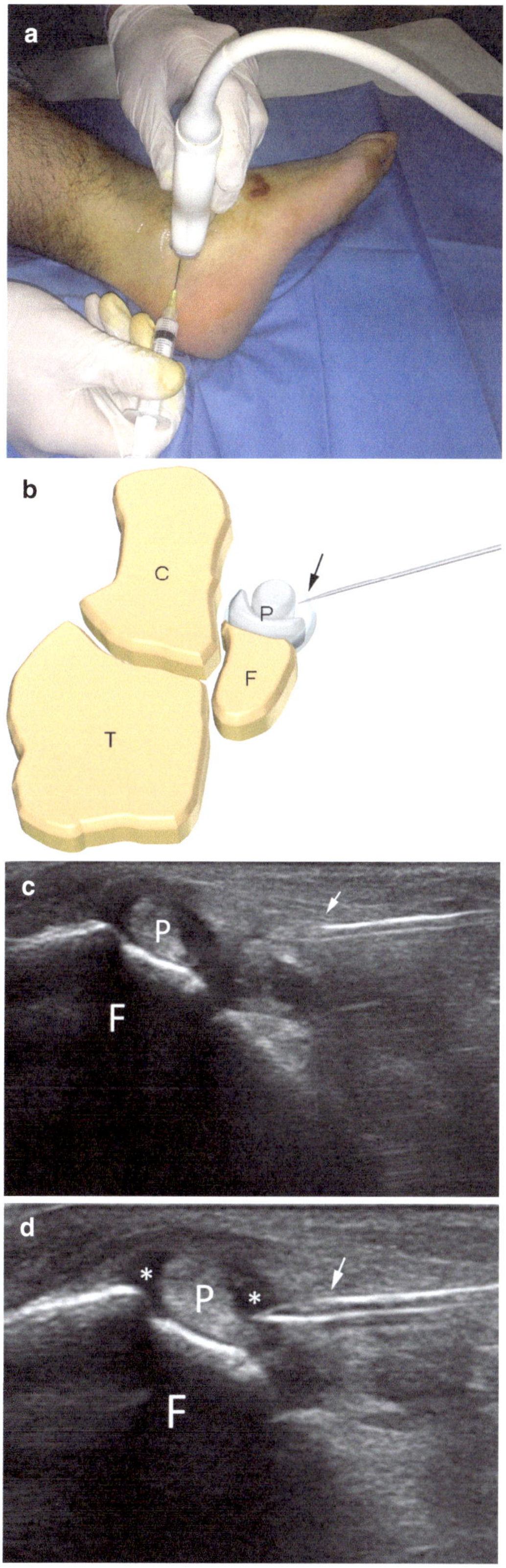

Fig. 16.1 US-guided treatment of peroneal tenosynovitis on a short axis. (**a**) Probe and patient position to perform US-guided treatment of peroneal tenosynovitis. (**b**) Anatomical scheme and (**c**) US image of needle insertion within peroneal tendon sheath, *C* calcaneus, *T* tibia, *F* fibula, *P* peroneal tendons, *arrow* needle tip. (**d**) Steroid injection (*asterisks*)

Part IV

The Foot

The Foot: Focused US Anatomy and Examination Technique

17

Davide Orlandi and Francesca Lacelli

The foot can be subdivided into the hindfoot and the forefoot. The hindfoot has a plantar side only, while the forefoot can be evaluated on both the dorsal and the plantar side.

Hindfoot

The patient lies supine or prone with the foot hanging out of the bed.

The foot must be dorsally flexed with the first toe extended. Then place the probe longitudinally over the heel to evaluate the insertional region of *plantar aponeurosis* on a longitudinal scan.

The plantar aponeurosis is generally considered as a modification of the deep fascia of the foot. It arises from the plantar aspect of the posteromedial calcaneal tuberosity and courses distally subdividing into central, medial, and lateral components. The medial band is the most commonly affected component (Fig. 17.1).

Forefoot, Plantar Side

The probe must be oriented on an axial plane over the metatarsal heads. At this level, the intermetatarsal spaces and flexor digitorum tendons can be seen.

Soft tissues within the intermetatarsal spaces must be evaluated displacing them from their natural position. This can be done either by pressing the skin on the dorsal side of the foot or by lateral squeezing of the whole forefoot (Mulder's maneuver). These maneuvers allow for an improved detection of intermetatarsal bursitis or Morton's neuroma.

Flexor tendons and metatarsophalangeal joints can be assessed using longitudinal scans and passive mobilization of toes. Dynamic scans allow also for detecting the integrity of plantar plates (Fig. 17.2).

D. Orlandi (✉)
Department of Internal Medicine,
University of Genova,
Genova, Italy
e-mail: theabo@libero.it

F. Lacelli
Unit of Radiology, Ospedale Santa Corona,
ASL 2 Savonese, Pietra Ligure, Italy
e-mail: lafrancy78@libero.it

L.M. Sconfienza et al. (eds.), *Ultrasound-guided Musculoskeletal Procedures: The Lower Limb*, DOI 10.1007/978-88-470-5764-7_17

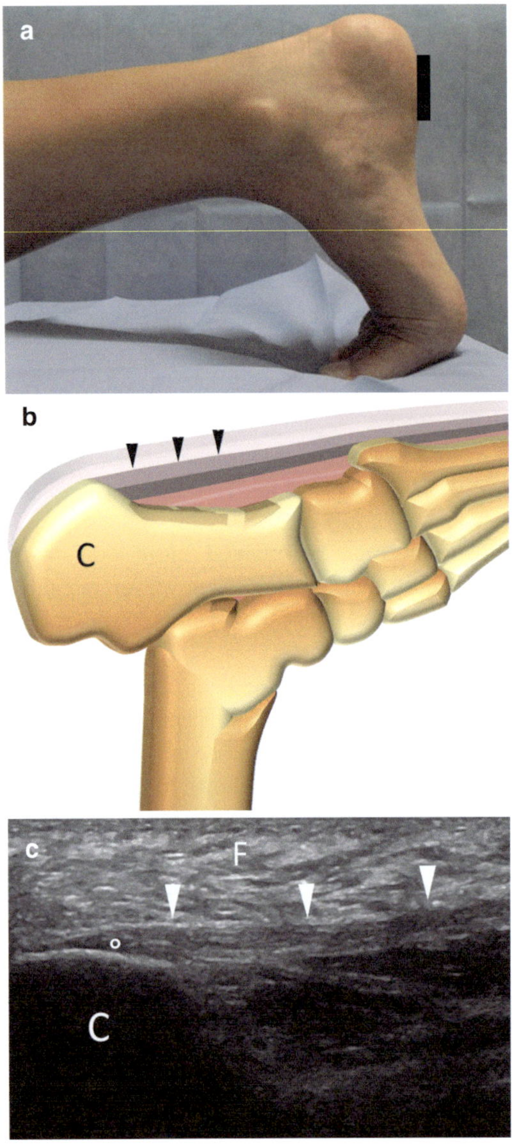

Fig. 17.1 Evaluation of the plantar hindfoot to assess the plantar fascia. (**a**) The probe and patient are positioned to evaluate the plantar fascia on a long-axis scan. (**b**) Anatomical scheme of the plantar fascia as seen along its long axis, *C* calcaneus. (**c**) US long-axis scan of the medial branch of the plantar fascia , *F fat pad, arrowheads medial branch of the plantar fascia, circles enthesis of the plantar fascia, partially affected by anisotropy artifacts*

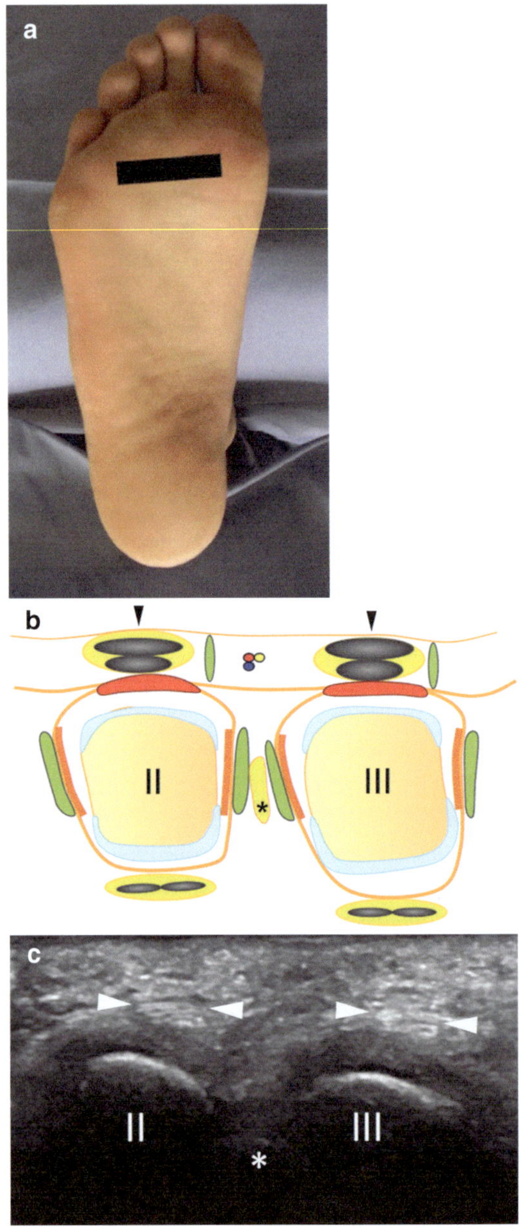

Fig. 17.2 Evaluation of the plantar forefoot to assess the intermetatarsal space. (**a**) The probe and patient are positioned to evaluate the intermetatarsal space on a short-axis scan. (**b**) Anatomical scheme of the intermetatarsal space as seen along its short axis, *II* 2nd metatarsal head, *III* 3rd metatarsal head, *arrowheads* flexor tendons, *asterisk* 2nd intermetatarsal space. (**c**) US short-axis scan of the intermetatarsal space

18 Plantar Fasciitis Dry-Needling Procedure

Davide Orlandi and Luca Maria Sconfienza

Essentials

Plantar fasciitis is the most common cause of inferior heel pain and may affect people who practice sport causing an overload on the hindfoot. It may also be associated with biomechanical factors such as pes cavus or foot pronation, with increased body weight, or with the presence of a calcaneal spur.

Epidemiology

Plantar fasciitis generally affects a wide range of individuals 40–60 years old, with equal prevalence among males and females.

D. Orlandi (✉)
Department of Internal Medicine,
University of Genova,
Genova, Italy
e-mail: theabo@libero.it

L.M. Sconfienza
Unit of Radiology, IRCCS Policlinico San Donato,
Milano, Italy

Department of Biomedical Sciences for Health,
University of Milano, Milano, Italy
e-mail: io@lucasconfienza.it

Clinical Presentation

Patients complain of a localized pain over the inferomedial aspect of the heel that worsens in the morning and is exacerbated by the conditions reported above. Often, symptoms persist for months or years and, if the pain is bilateral, it could be the consequence of systemic conditions like rheumatologic or metabolic affections.

Diagnosis

In most cases, imaging is not necessary since the diagnosis of plantar fasciitis is usually made on a clinical basis. Imaging can be used to evaluate the extent of tissue damage; to exclude other causes of heel pain, when the clinical presentation is atypical; or to confirm the diagnosis in patients not responding to conservative treatment. Plain radiographs may depict the presence of a calcaneal spur or be normal. Magnetic resonance imaging and ultrasound can be useful to confirm the diagnosis.

Treatment Options

Plantar fasciitis treatment is usually conservative and relies on restriction of physical activity, NSAIDs, and physical therapy with elongation

L.M. Sconfienza et al. (eds.), *Ultrasound-guided Musculoskeletal Procedures: The Lower Limb*, DOI 10.1007/978-88-470-5764-7_18

exercises. Shockwave therapy can reduce symptoms in the middle term. Surgical debridement or fasciotomy is reserved for refractory cases. US-guided scarification (dry needling) can be considered as a minimally invasive option.

Interventional Procedure

Indications

Insertional or pre-insertional overload fasciopathy of the medial o lateral branch of the plantar aponeurosis. Contraindicated in case of traumatic lesions of the plantar aponeurosis

How We Do It

Objective

To cause local hyperemia and bleeding into the plantar aponeurosis, thus promoting post-procedural platelet-induced recovery phenomena

Equipment

- 1 syringe (5 ml)
- 1 syringe (2 ml)
- 25G needle
- 20G spinal needle
- Lidocaine (5–10 ml)
- Long-acting steroid (1 ml, 40 mg/ml)
- Plaster

STEP 1
The patient lies supine or prone with the foot hanging out of the bed with the ankle flexed 90°. The plantar aponeurosis is seen on an axial scan, starting from the calcaneal insertion and moving the probe caudally to identify the level of more severe affection. The 25G needle is inserted in the medial aspect of the heel with an in-plane approach, in a medial-lateral direction. Anesthetic is injected along the path of the needle, in the peritendinous soft tissues, and in the degenerated portion of the plantar aponeurosis (Fig. 18.1).

STEP 2
With the same needle used for anesthesia, a number of punctures is performed within the thickened portion of the fascia. Usually, 10 to 20 punctures are sufficient for a good result.

STEP 3
Complete the procedure injecting one ml of steroid into the perifascial soft tissues, deep to the fascial insertion, avoiding the plantar aponeurosis and the plantar fat pad. The needle is then removed and a plaster applied.

Post-procedural Care
The patient is kept under observation for about 10 min. Pain may occur after treatment and is managed with oral NSAIDs. Patients are advised to use an orthotic support and to reduce their physical activity, although no systematic rest period is suggested.

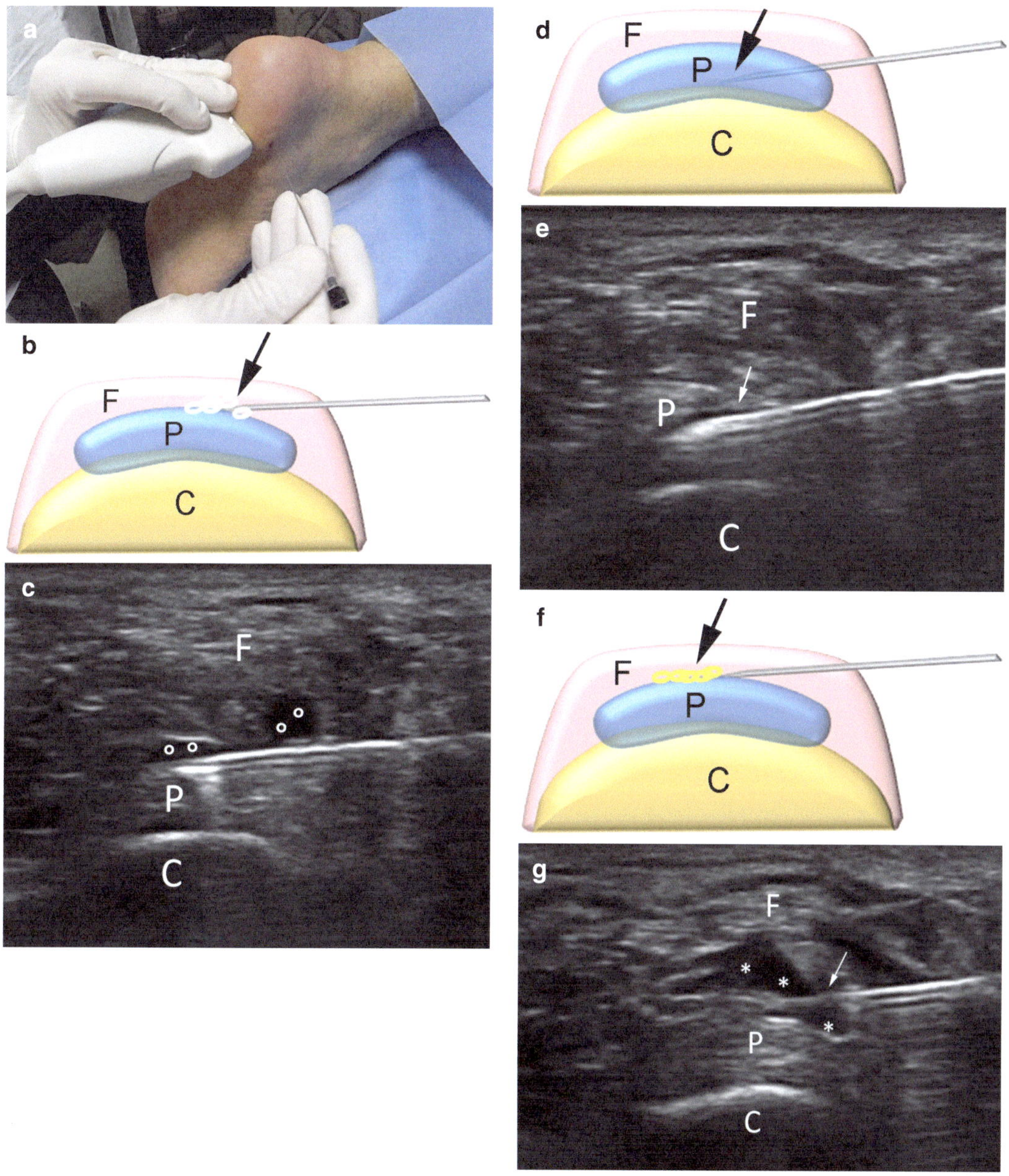

Fig. 18.1 US-guided treatment of plantar fasciitis on a short-axis scan. (**a**) Probe and patient position to perform short-axis US-guided treatment of plantar fasciitis. (**b**) Anatomical scheme and (**c**) US scan of anesthetic injection around the plantar fascia, *F* fat pat, *P* plantar fascia, *C* calcaneus, *circle* anesthetic, *arrow* needle tip. (**d**) Anatomical scheme and (**e**) US scan of dry-needling procedure. (**f**) Anatomical scheme and (**g**) US scan of steroid injection (*asterisks*) over the plantar fascia

Treatment of Morton's Neuroma and Intermetatarsal Bursitis

19

Angelo Corazza and Riccardo Sartoris

Essentials

Morton's metatarsalgia is an uncommon painful condition of the forefoot affecting the plantar side usually between the third and fourth toes. This condition could be sustained by a neuroma (Morton's neuroma) rather by an intermetatarsal bursitis.

Morton's neuroma is a swollen nerve in the ball of the foot, commonly between the base of the second and third toes.

Although labeled as a neuroma, histological studies demonstrate that it is not a true tumor, but rather a perineural fibrosis (fibrous tissue formation around nerve tissue).

Etiology and Clinical Presentation

Morton's neuroma may be the result of irritation, pressure, or injury. High percentage of patients with Morton's neuroma is women who wear high-heeled or narrow shoes.

This condition is basically an entrapment syndrome causing a sharp burning pain in the ball of the foot. There may also be numbness, burning, and stinging in the toes.

Morton's neuroma signs and symptoms, which usually occur unexpectedly and tend to worsen over time, include pain on weight bearing and shooting pain affecting the contiguous halves of two toes.

Sometimes there may be a dull pain rather than a sharp one. Typically, a patient will suddenly experience pain while walking and will have to stop and remove their shoe.

Diagnosis

In most cases, the diagnosis of Morton's metatarsalgia is made on a clinical basis. Imaging can be used to confirm the diagnosis in patients not responding to conservative treatment. Ultrasound can help to detect the presence of an intermetatarsal neuroma, but sometimes the differential diagnosis with a chronic intermetatarsal bursitis could be challenging. Magnetic resonance imaging can be useful to confirm the diagnosis and sometimes require the use of paramagnetic contrast in order to differentiate the perineural edema from the real neuroma.

A. Corazza (✉) • R. Sartoris
Postgraduate School in Radiodiagnostics,
University of Genova, School of
Medicine, Genova, Italy
e-mail: angelcoraz@libero.it;
riccardo.sartoris@hotmail.it

L.M. Sconfienza et al. (eds.), *Ultrasound-guided Musculoskeletal Procedures: The Lower Limb*, DOI 10.1007/978-88-470-5764-7_19

Treatment Options

Patients with Morton's neuroma may need to change their footwear and take painkillers. Steroid injections could be useful in order to treat the intermetatarsal bursitis, while neuromas may require injections. Surgery is reserved for refractory cases in order to either remove the affected nerve or release the pressure on it.

Interventional Procedure

Indications

Forefoot pain caused by Morton's neuroma or intermetatarsal bursitis. This treatment has no real contraindications.

Objective

To inject anti-inflammatory drugs/alcohol into the intermetatarsal space to treat intermetatarsal pain

Equipment

- 1 syringe (2 ml)
- 25G needle
- Lidocaine (2 ml) + long-acting steroid (1 ml, 40 mg/ml)
- Lidocaine (4 ml) + 95 % ethylic alcohol (1–2 ml)
- Plaster

How We Do It

STEP 1

The patient lies supine on the bed. To reach the intermetatarsal space, different approaches can be used. The probe can be placed on axial scan over the plantar aspect of the metatarsal heads to visualize the pertinent intermetatarsal space. The needle is then inserted with coaxial (out-plane) approach. Only the needle tip will be seen. Alternatively, the probe can be positioned between the two fingers with sagittal orientation and the needle can be inserted with a lateral (in-plane) approach from the dorsum of the foot. This latter approach allows for a better visualization of needle track.

STEP 2

Intermetatarsal bursitis: the needle tip is inserted in the bursa and 1 ml of anesthetic and 1 ml of long-lasting steroid is injected within the bursa.

Morton's neuroma: there is no consensus regarding which is the best treatment for this pathology. We initially prefer to use a mixture of 2+1 ml of anesthetic and steroid injected around the neuroma. In case of treatment failure after 1 month, we perform a second procedure using 4 ml of anesthetic and 1–2 ml of 95 % ethylic alcohol with the same technique. Note that alcohol injection is particularly painful, so a generous amount of anesthesia should be injected priory (Fig. 19.1).

STEP 3

The needle is removed and a plaster applied.

Post-procedural Care

The patient is kept under observation for at about 10 min. Pain may occur after treatment and is managed with oral NSAIDs. Patients are advised to use an orthotic support to relieve the forefoot, although no systematic rest period is suggested.

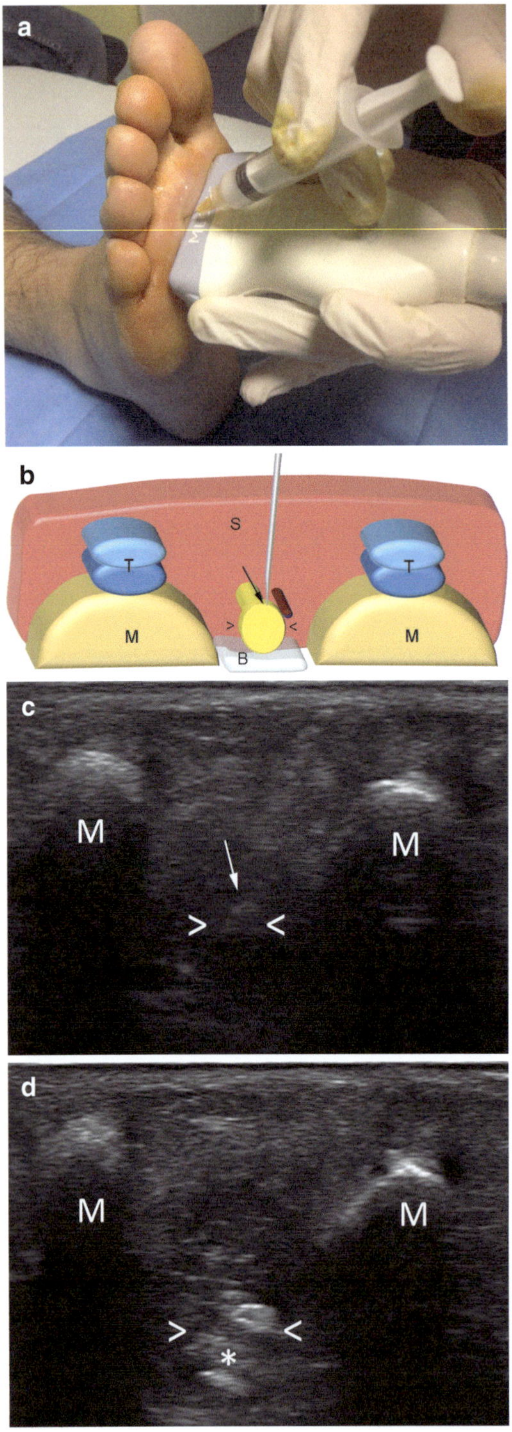

Fig. 19.1 US-guided treatment of Morton's neuroma with coaxial approach. (**a**) Probe and patient position to perform US-guided treatment of Morton's neuroma. (**b**) Anatomical scheme and (**c**) US image of perineural needle insertion, *M* metatarsal heads, *T* flexor tendons, *S* subcutaneous tissue, *arrow* needle tip, *arrowheads* neuroma, *B* intermetatarsal bursa. (**d**) Steroid injection (*asterisk*)

MIX
Papier aus verantwortungsvollen Quellen
Paper from responsible sources
FSC® C105338

If you have any concerns about our products,
you can contact us on
ProductSafety@springernature.com

In case Publisher is established outside the EU,
the EU authorized representative is:
Springer Nature Customer Service Center GmbH
Europaplatz 3, 69115 Heidelberg, Germany

Printed by Libri Plureos GmbH
in Hamburg, Germany